Traditional Meniscectomy

Single Surgical Procedures **2**

A Colour Atlas of

Traditional Meniscectomy

I. S. Smillie

W DE G

Walter de Gruyter · Berlin · New York 1984

Ian S. Smillie OBE, Ch. M, FRCS (Ed.), FRCS (Glas.); Sometime Professor of Orthopaedic Surgery, University of St. Andrews; Emeritus Professor of Orthopaedic Surgery, University of Dundee; President of the International Society of the Knee

Original Publishers: Wolfe Medical Publications Ltd., · London
Exclusive co-publishers for the Federal Republic of Germany and Austria: Walter de Gruyter & Co., Genthiner Strasse 13, D-1000 Berlin 30. 1984.

Printed by Royal Smeets Offset b. v., Weert, Netherlands

Cover design: Rudolf Hübler

General Editor, Wolfe Surgical Atlases:
William F. Walker, DSc, ChM, FRCS (Eng.), FRCS (Edin.), FRS (Edin.)

CIP-Kurztitelaufnahme der Deutschen Bibliothek

Smillie, Ian S.:
A colour atlas of traditional meniscectomy / I. S. Smillie. –
Berlin; New York: de Gruyter, 1984.
(Single surgical procedures; 2)
ISBN 3-11-010009-6
ISBN 3-11-010008-8 (Subskr.-Pr.)
NE: GT

Contents

Introduction

The operation of meniscectomy, the commonest performed in orthopaedic surgery, is one of simplicity or, alternatively, fraught with technical difficulties even in the most expert hands. All in all it appears to pose problems for the average surgeon. It is the operation I am asked to perform for visitors. It is the only operation I am asked to demonstrate overseas.

It is an operation which depends for success on 'know-how' at every step. It is the object of this monograph to describe the 'know-how'. The operation to be described depends on the use of knives (meniscotomes) to my design to achieve total meniscectomy through a limited exposure. The design was finalised in 1939 and has not been modified in any respect since then.

I am frequently asked what prompted my interest in the knee joint, in the pathology of the menisci, and meniscectomy in particular. When the Orthopaedic Department of the Royal Infirmary of Edinburgh was inaugurated in 1936 and I became Clinical Assistant to Mr Walter Mercer, later Professor Sir Walter, I noted a certain reluctance on the part of patients to accept surgery as a solution to problems of internal derangement relative to a meniscus. All had friends or relatives subjected to operations whose knees no longer locked but who were not cured in so far as the joint remained unstable. They were not impressed by the results of surgery as then performed. The reason soon became clear: none of the surgeons for whom I worked could perform a total meniscectomy. Failure to remove the posterior segment was the reason for the dissatisfaction. Here was a challenge: design instruments for total excision. I found at an early stage of development that you could not push a knife into a joint in one direction and expect it to cut in another. All the modifications of 'Smillie's knives', of which three are illustrated, attempt to do just that. The curves of the knives cannot be increased without revealing total ignorance of their mode of use.

There are three knives. The one in the centre (see **1**) is no more than a miniature chisel. It is intended to be passed, blade vertical, between the periphery of the meniscus about its mid point and the long fibres of the medial ligament. It is the least important of the three in that a scalpel can perform the same function.

The other two, right and left, consist of a curved cutting edge between blunt points of different length, the longer of which lies on the tibial table. The terminal three centimetres or so is gently curved. The knives are used at an angle of 45 degrees to the vertical; and this is the reason why the curve cannot be increased.

Finally, after the meniscus is dislocated into the intercondylar notch, is shown the semi-diagrammatic method of division of the postero-central attachment whereby the longer beak of one of the curved knives is placed underneath the meniscus and division effected by backward pressure.

The exact dimensions of the knives are of importance. So many distortions, but particularly enlargements, of the instruments are on sale in world markets, and presented to me to use as my own abroad, that in my defence, and in the hope of better things, engineers' drawings were published (Smillie, 1978). Alas, without any noticeable improvement. Instrument manufacturers do not consult surgical monographs.

The importance of these meniscotomes and their mode of use has determined that pride of place should be given to them in the detailed description of the steps of meniscectomy.

I have no vested interest in these knives other than the wish to instruct in their exact mode of use in the manner intended. It is suggested therefore that several sets of the curved models be available when a meniscectomy is performed. If the surgeon is given a blunt knife others, hopefully sharp, are available.

It is well known that instruments designed for one purpose are found to be equally useful for another. It is relevant to interpose at this point, that in the anterior compartment syndrome the deep fascia can be split with a curved knife through an incision little bigger than a stab wound. In a similar fashion the lateral capsular expansion at the knee can be divided in the so-called 'lateral release' operation. In the carpal tunnel syndrome the transverse carpal ligament can be divided with a curved knife.

Meniscotomes

1 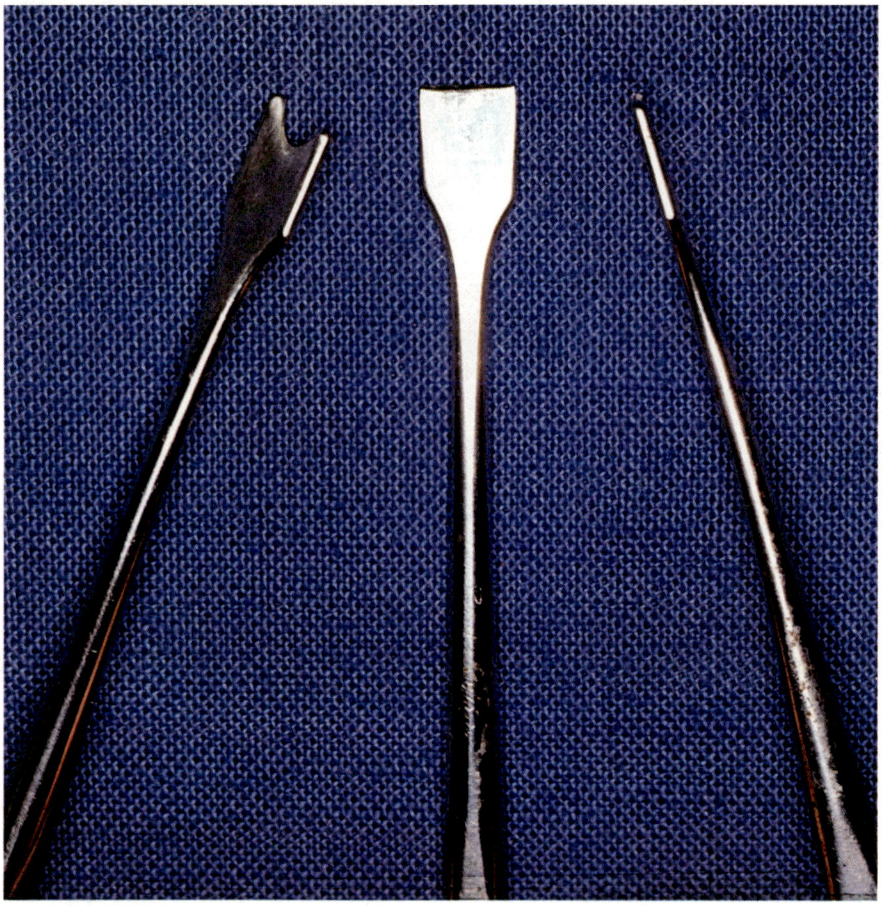

1 The knives (meniscotomes). The operation to be described depends on the use of special meniscus knives. In the centre is the chisel knife intended to be passed, the blade vertical, between the centre of the periphery and the collateral ligament. The two curved knives, right and left, consist of a blade enclosed between blunt beaks. In use the long beak lies on the tibial head. The gentle curve involves the terminal 2.5 to 3cm and enables them to be used at 45 degrees to the vertical (see **2** and **3**) where they take up the minimal space within the joint.

2

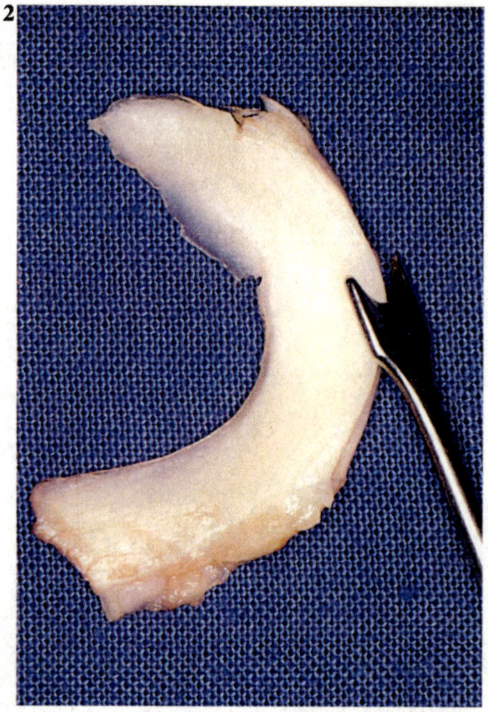

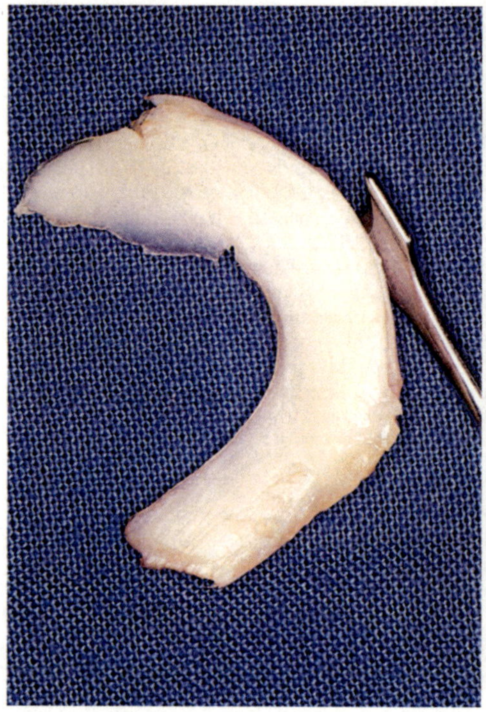

2 The knives: mode of use (semi-diagrammatic). Right lateral meniscus is mobilised by division of the peripheral synovial attachments with the knife rotated 45 degrees towards the centre of the joint. The attachments are divided under tension by traction exerted by the Martin's forceps (not shown).

3 The knives: modes of use (semi-diagrammatic). Left lateral meniscus mobilised by division of the synovial attachments with the knife rotated 45 degrees towards the periphery. The attachments are divided under tension by traction exerted by the Martin's forceps 22 (not shown).

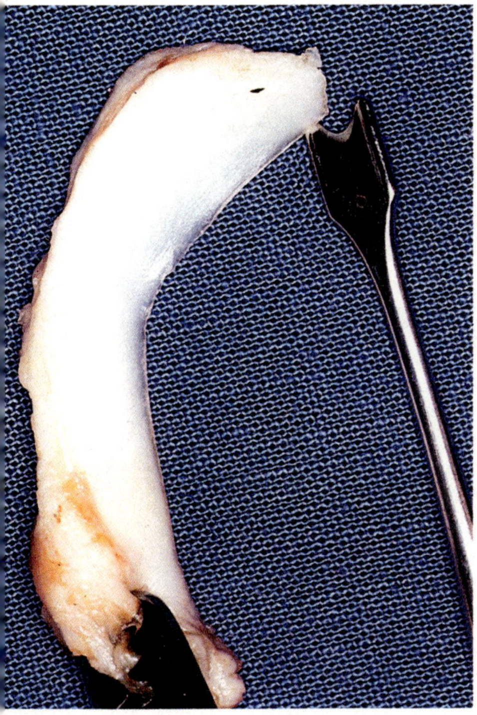

5

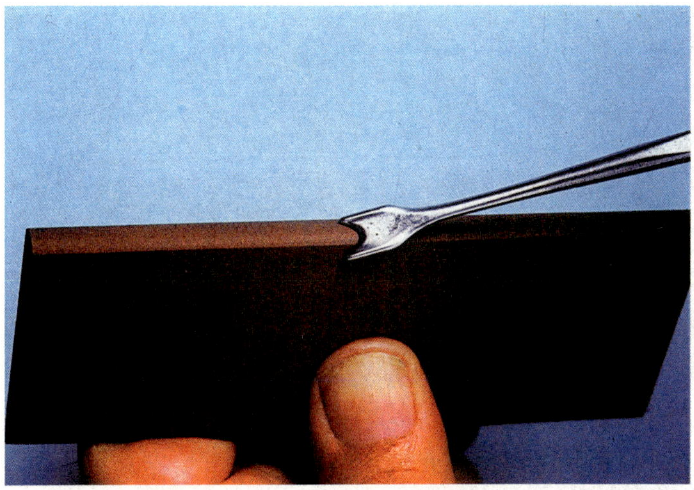

5 The knives: maintenance. It is essential that the cutting edges be kept sharp; and a special hone is available to this end. It is dangerous to be required to use force with a blunt knife. The flat side of the hone is used on the chisel knife. The rounded margin on the curved knives.

4 The knives: mode of use (semi-diagrammatic). The final action in meniscectomy is division of the postero-central attachment after the meniscus has been dislocated into the centre of the joint. This is accomplished, using the appropriate curved knife, by placing the long beak beneath the postero-central attachment and with the meniscus under tension, pushing the knife directly backwards.

6

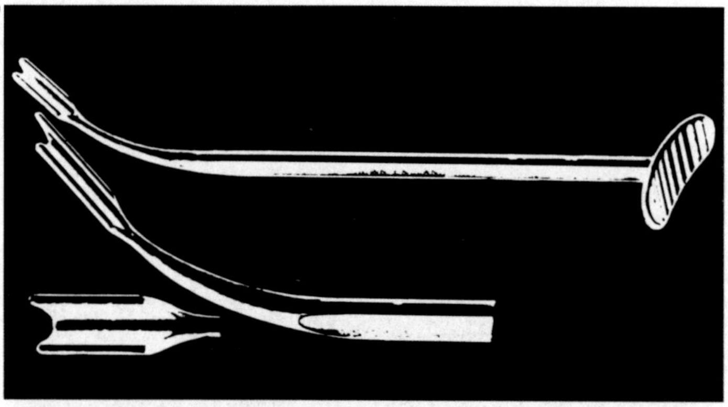

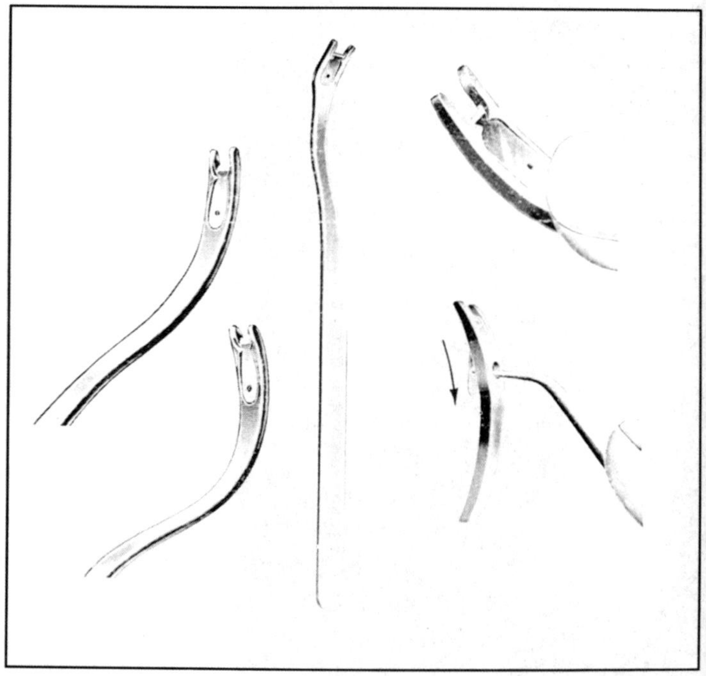

8

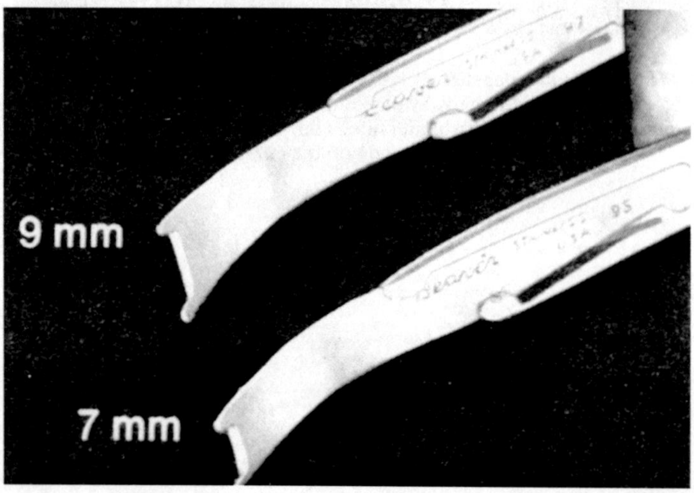

6, 7 and 8 Meniscotomes. Numerous meniscotomes are available on the market, based on my design, of which three are illustrated here. They seek by greatly increasing the curve of the blade, to improve on the originals. The Introduction states that it was discovered at an early stage of development that you cannot push a knife into a joint in one direction and expect it to cut in another. To increase the curve of the knives is to fail to understand their mode of action.

Draining the limb

9

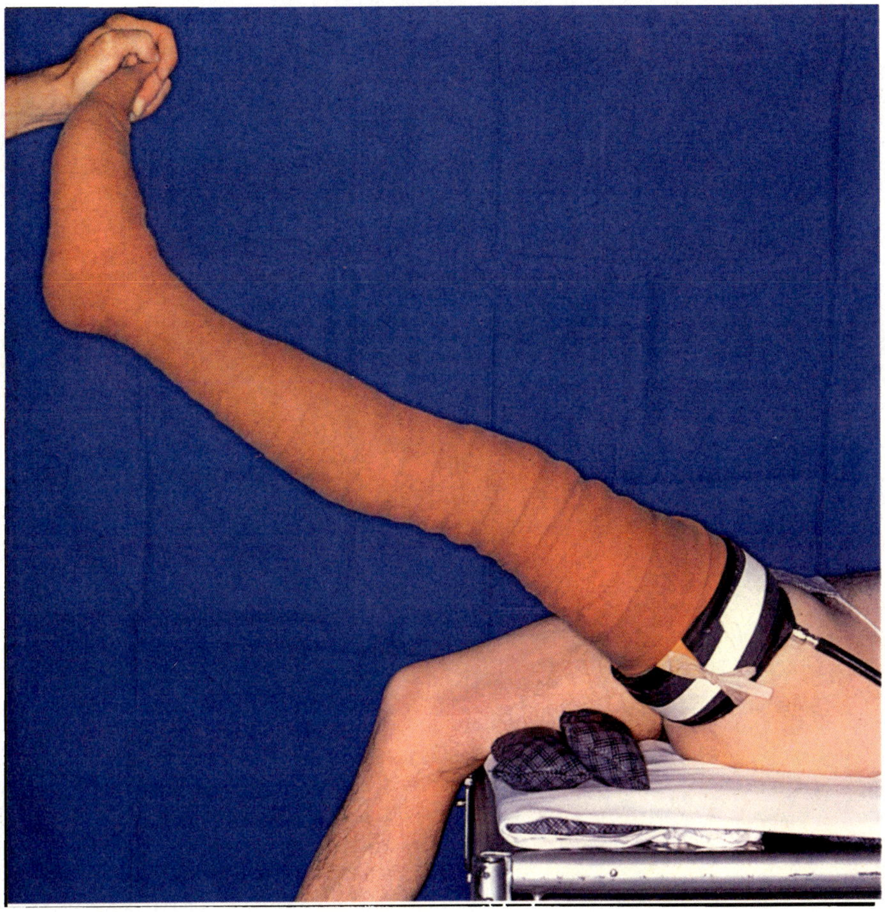

9 **Meniscectomy step by step.** The limb is drained with an elastic (Esmarch) bandage and the pneumatic tourniquet inflated. Note sandbag beneath thigh. Note also that the end of the operating table has been removed.

10 Position on table. The sandbag beneath the thigh can with advantage be triangular in section. The knee is prepared and the antiseptic of choice applied in extension.

10

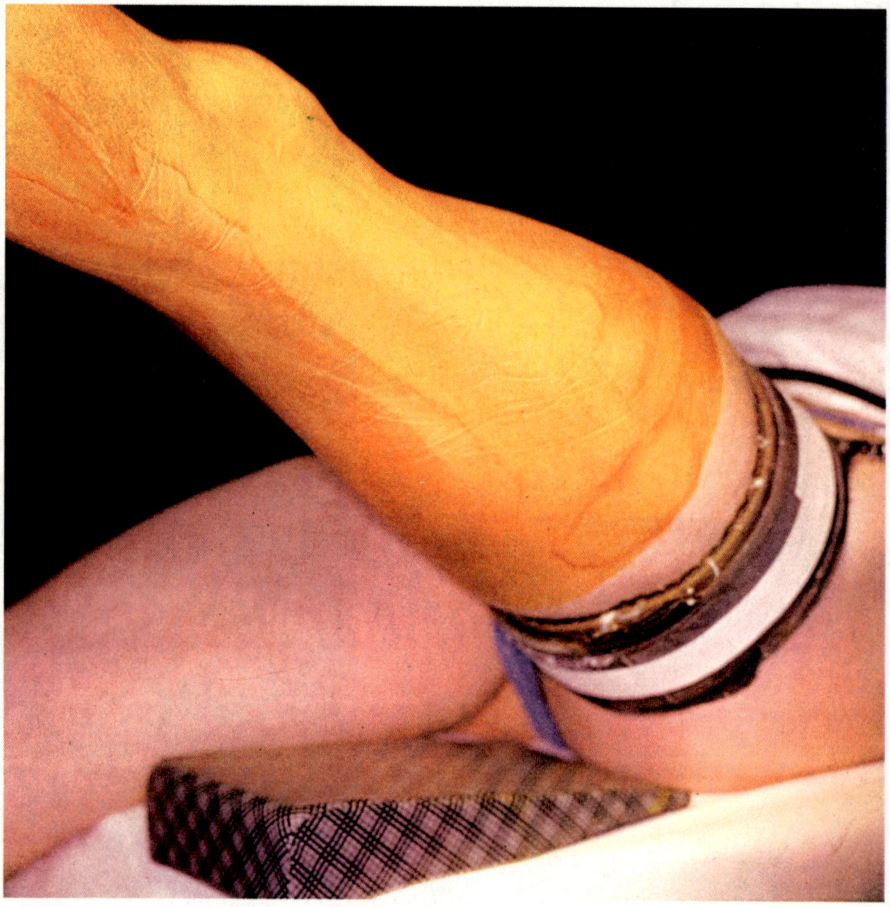

11 Re-apply antiseptic in flexion. When the joint is flexed the white creases indicate that the antiseptic has not penetrated and should be re-applied.

11

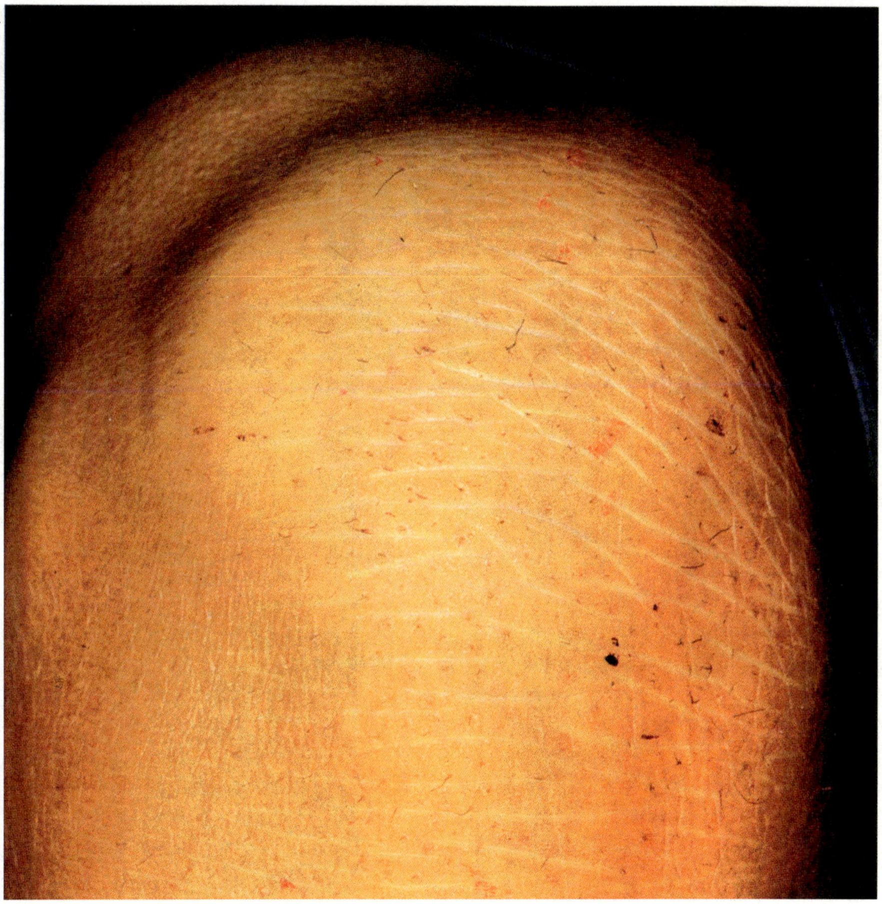

Position of surgeon

12

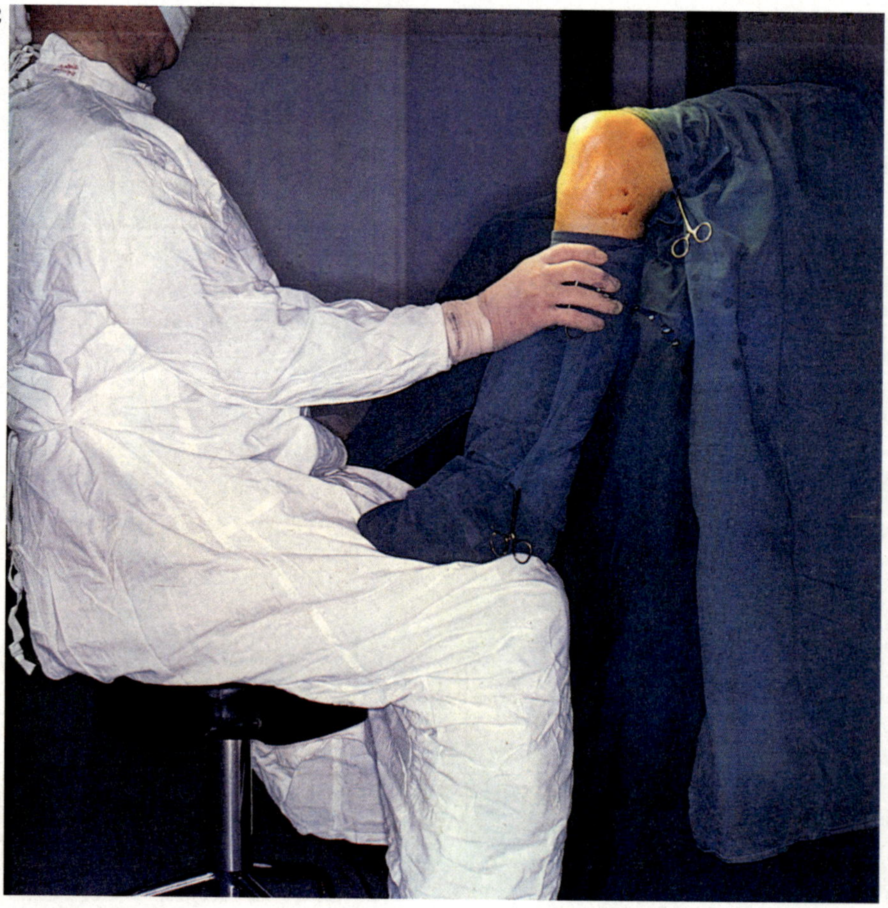

12 Position of surgeon. The height of the operating table is adjusted so that the surgeon's knees grip the patient's foot to produce lateral rotation of the tibia at the critical phase of the operation. To this end the surgeon's gown should be long so that in the action no lapse of aseptic technique can occur.

13 Popliteal structures to be mobile. The knee must hang clear of the table and the sandbag beneath the thigh so located that the popliteal structures are not fixed. If they are free, even if a meniscus knife slipped at a critical stage of the operation, they would probably escape injury. In no circumstances should the operation be performed with the knee flexed over a large wedge-shaped cushion.

13

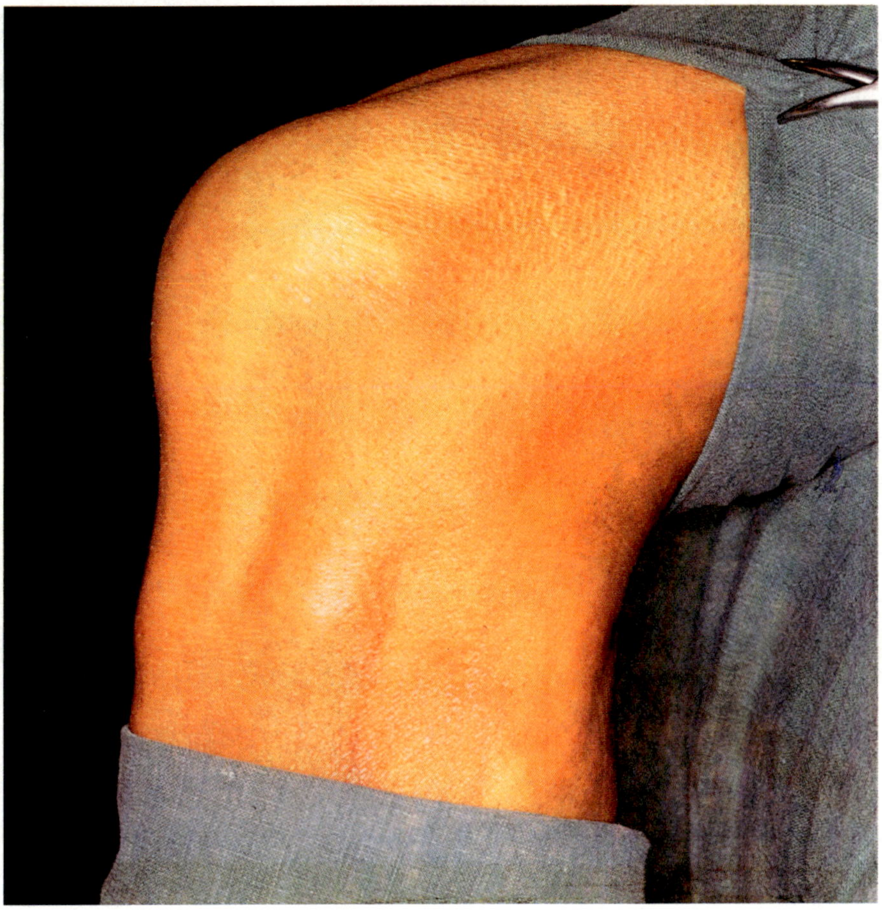

Incision site

14 Site of incision. The incision on the medial side should not extend more than a finger's breadth below the joint line, lest the infrapatellar branch of the saphenous nerve be endangered.

14

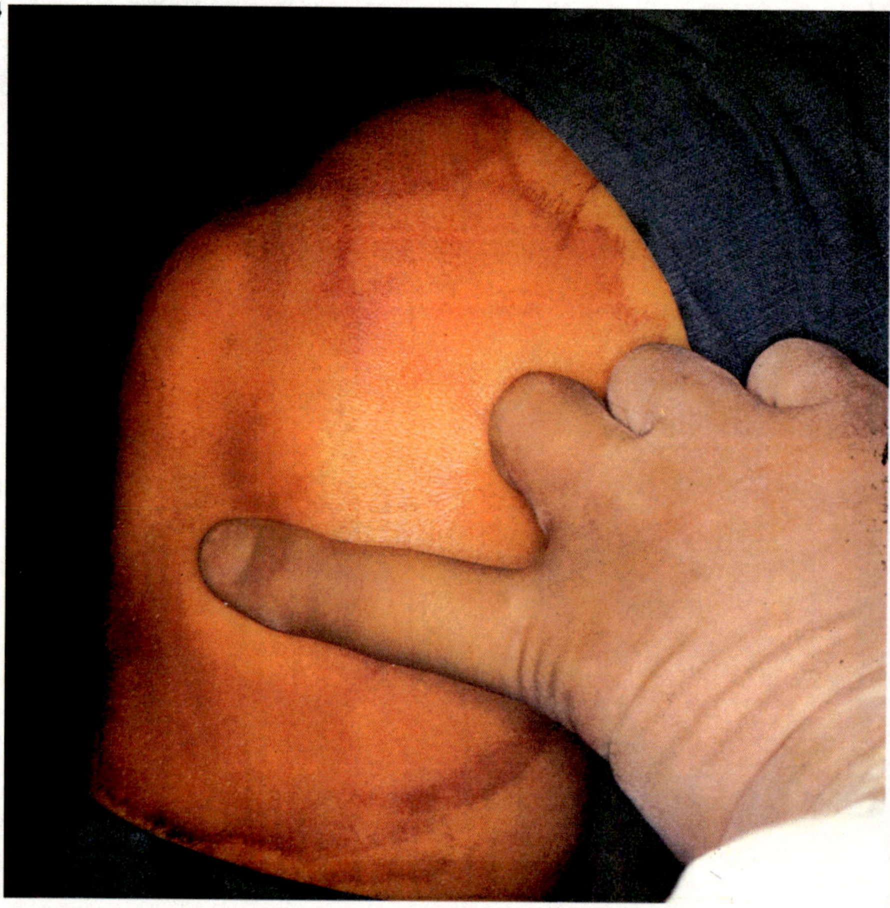

15 Site of incision. The location of the incision is important if the maximum access is to be obtained through a limited exposure. It is made through alcohol-soaked muslin, stockinette or other cloth material and begins at or about the junction of the broad upper-third of the patella with the inferior two-thirds.

15

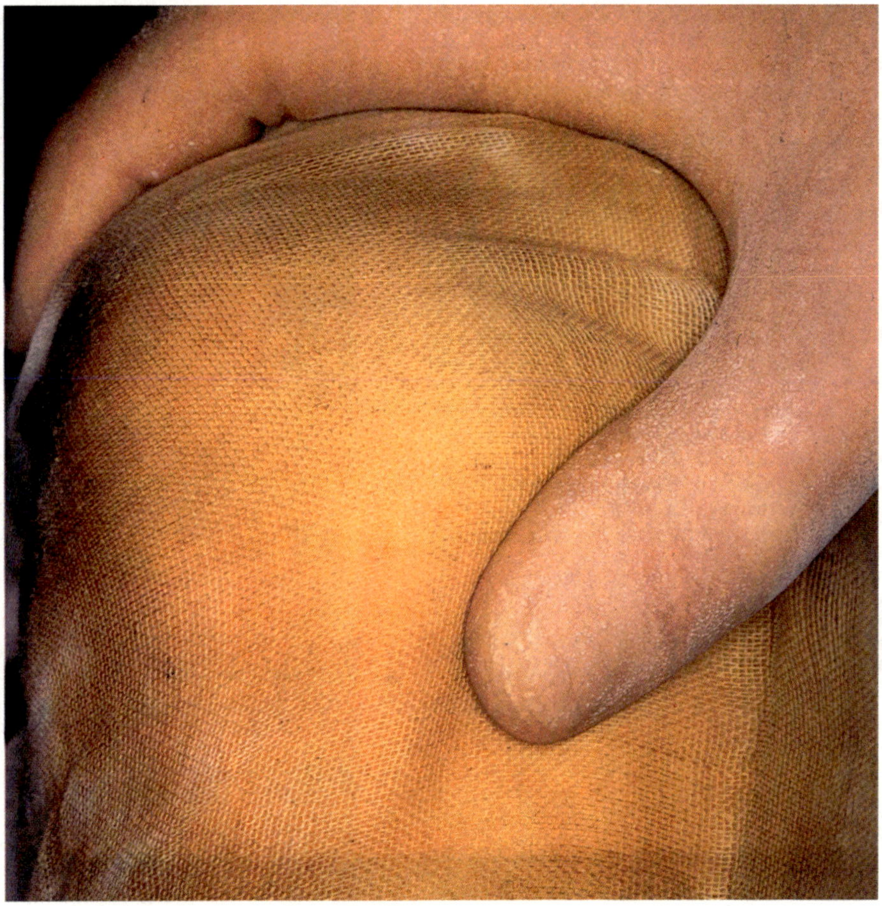

16 Site of incision. It extends downwards and slightly backwards to terminate not more than a finger's breadth below the joint line lest, as has been indicated, the infrapatellar branch of the saphenous nerve be endangered. On the lateral side the inferior limit of the skin incision is not critical.

Transverse incisions should be avoided because they prejudice healing of any future vertical incision. Vertical incisions which slope forwards rather than backwards provide less comfortable access to the posterior third of the meniscus at the most difficult part of the operation. The divided cloth material is turned over and clipped to the margins of the wound with light-weight Allis tissue forceps or Michel clips in such a manner that the edges are completely covered. Adhesive skin covering is not recommended in such a short incision in that the potentially dangerous skin edges, over which instruments will be passed, are not covered.

The scalpel used to make the skin incision is discarded.

16

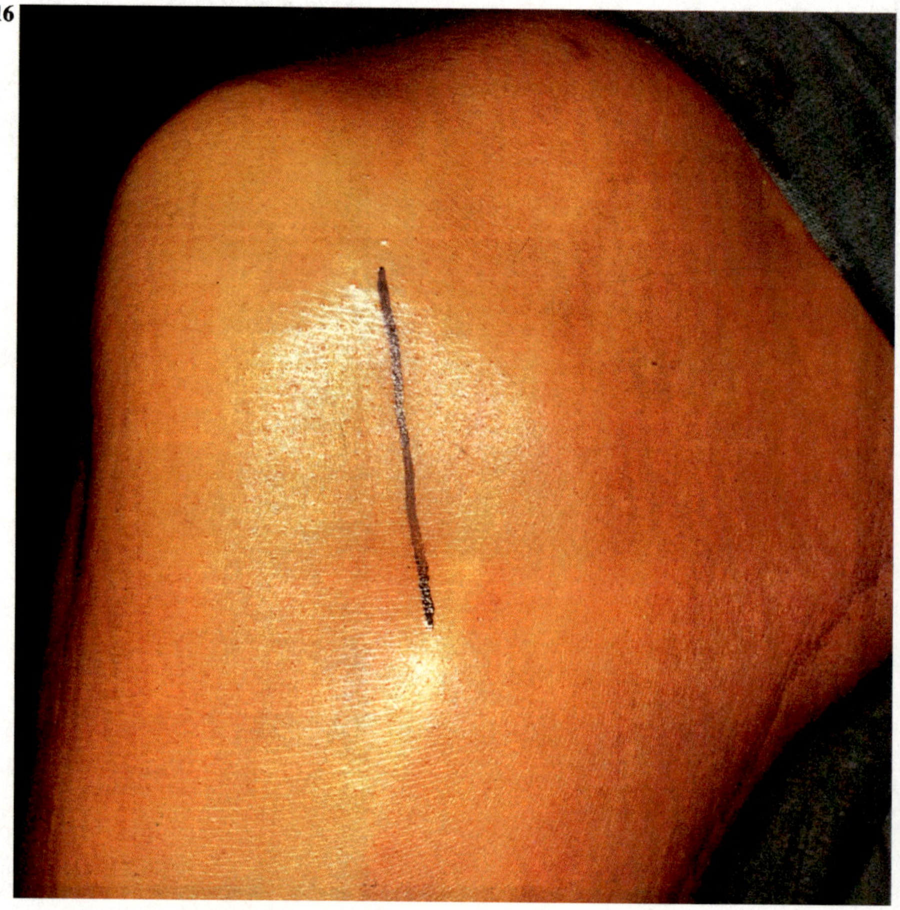

Capsule division

17 Division of capsule. The capsule is divided in the line of the skin incision using a fresh scalpel and exposing the extra synovial fat. The extra synovial fat and synovial membrane are divided vertically down to but not damaging the superior surface of the periphery of the meniscus. Retractors (**24**) are inserted to permit inspection of the interior of the joint. If it is a displaced bucket-handle tear the central portion will be immediately evident. If it is the more common horizontal cleavage lesion, nothing will be seen unless a flap from the undersurface of the posterior half has been displaced centrally. If it is a bucket-handle tear, decide before proceeding further whether the displaced portion only is to be removed or the entire meniscus excised. If the former action is selected the anterior horn must not be mobilised but the displaced portion divided at the limits of the tear anteriorly and posteriorly with one of the curved knives (**2** and **3**).

17

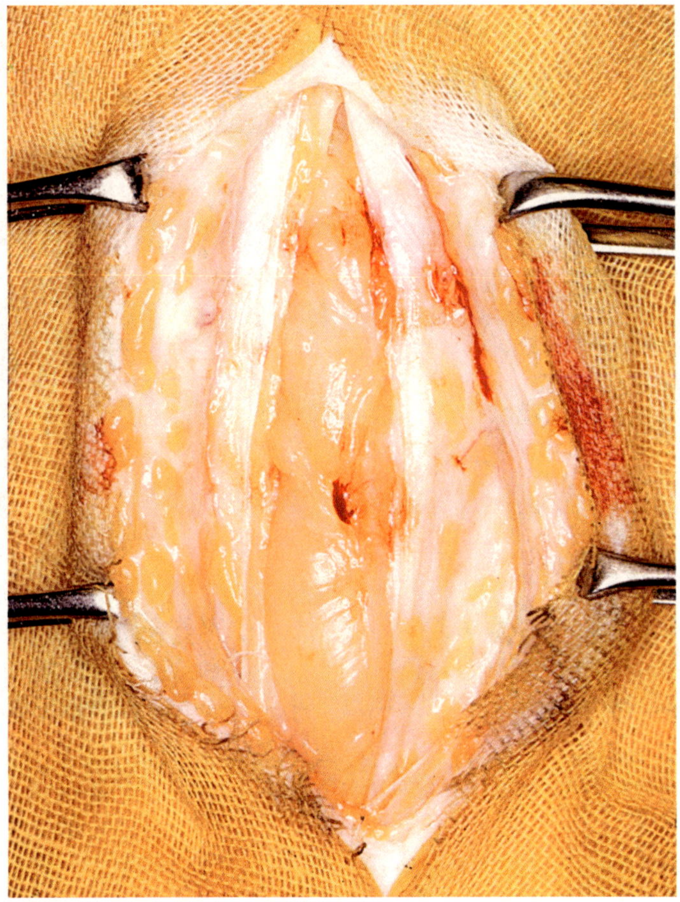

18

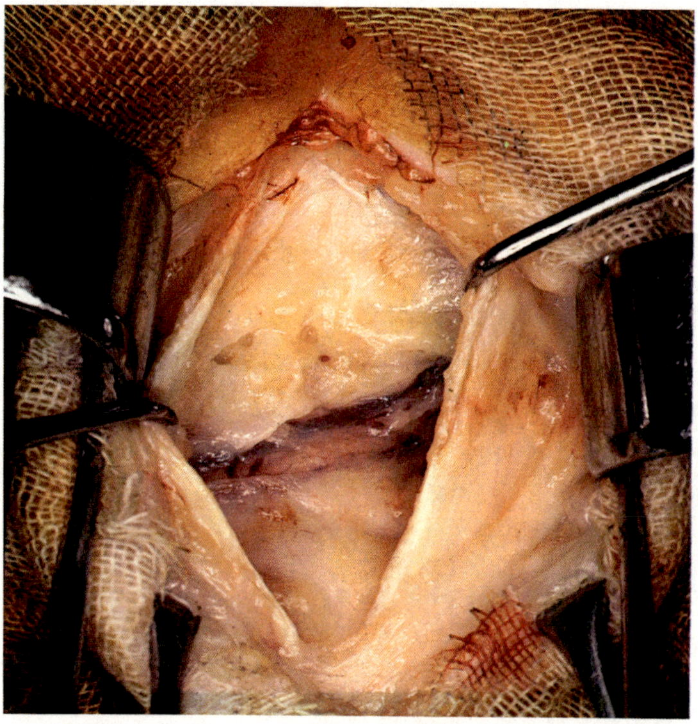

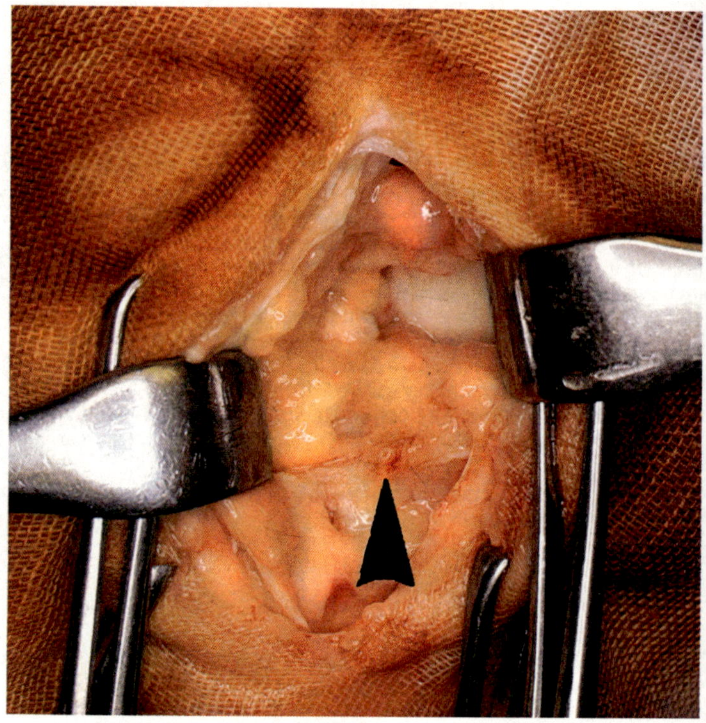

18 Avoiding postoperative haematoma. Subcapsular veins as large as these require ligation or coagulation.

19 Avoiding postoperative haematoma. In the bloodless field provided by the tourniquet arteries in the extra synovial fat, the lumen of which can be seen, require ligation or coagulation.

20 Dividing antero-central attachment. If it is decided to excise the entire meniscus, the anterior horn is lifted off the tibial head with toothed dissecting forceps and a horizontal incision made between the undersurface of meniscus and tibial head. It is now possible to locate the antero-central attachment which is divided close to the midline.

20

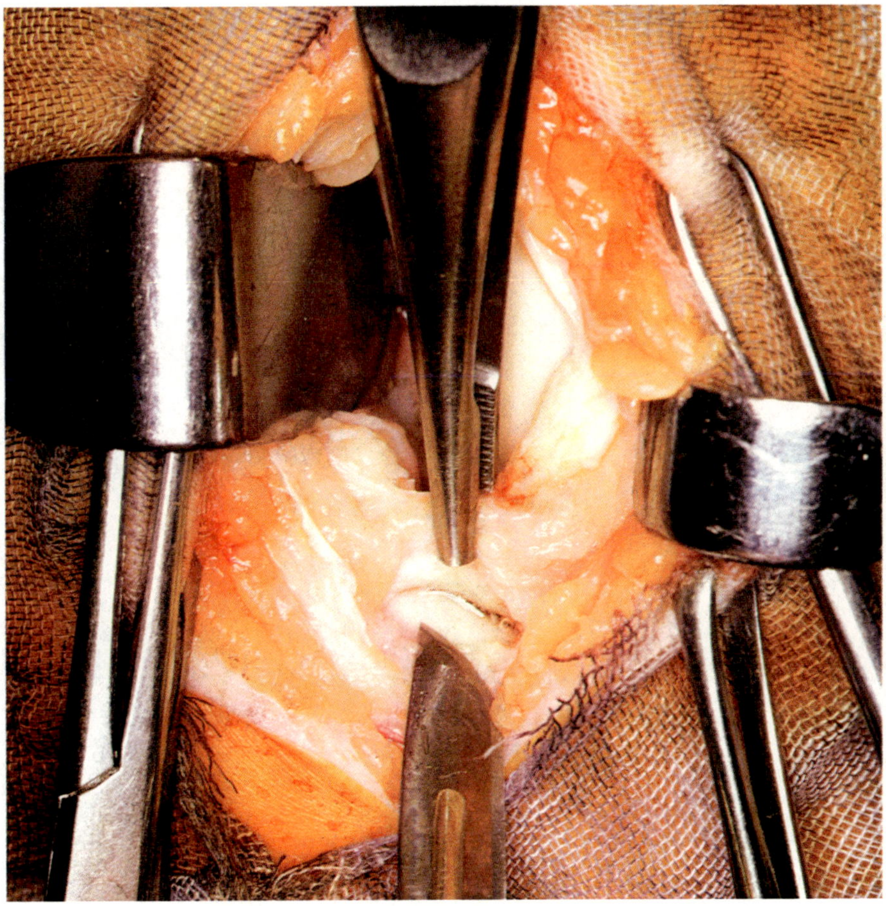

Defining meniscus

21 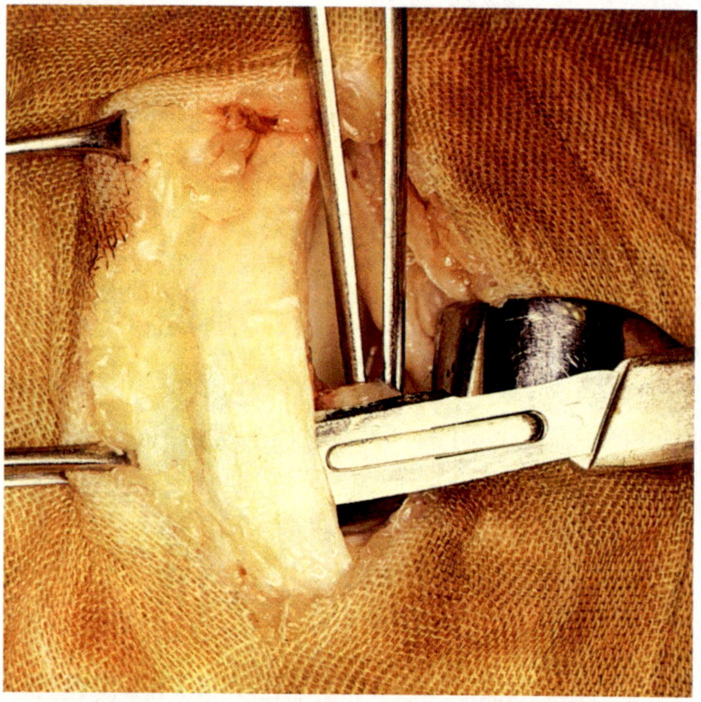

22 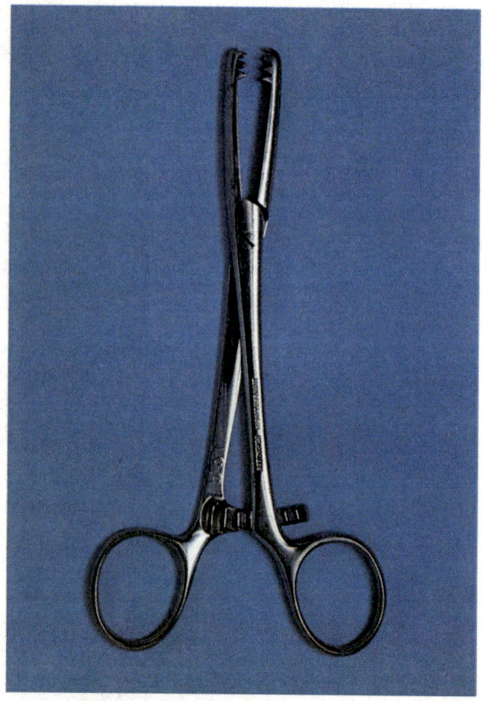

21 Defining the periphery of meniscus. The next move is to define the periphery of the meniscus. It is in doing so that the first serious error can occur in the uninitiated: with a retractor (**24**) exerting traction on the capsule it is very easy to cut into the periphery of the meniscus. Both retractors are therefore removed thus relaxing the capsule completely. With the anterior horn of the meniscus held with toothed dissecting forceps, the blade of the lightly held scalpel picks up the soft line of cleavage between periphery of meniscus and capsule.

22 Meniscus clamp. Excision of the meniscus demands, from the nature of the tissue involved, a special clamp to ensure the grip is maintained when traction is exerted. 'Martin's meniscus forceps' has square-cut teeth which grip the fibro-cartilage firmly. The total length should be limited to say 15cm, so that the hand so accommodated does not obscure the vision of the surgeon.

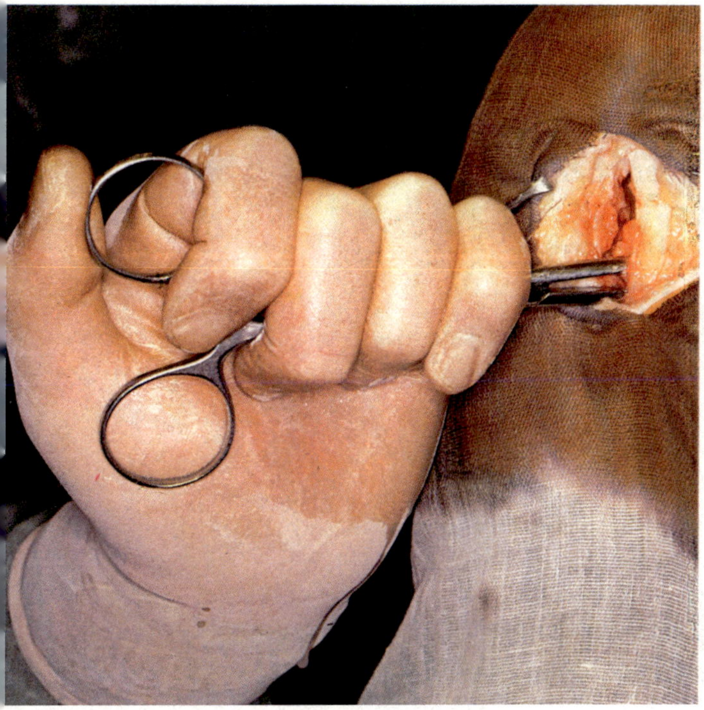

23 **Meniscus clamp: mode of use.** It is at this stage, and not before, that the meniscus clamp is applied. It is attached to the convex margin, not to the concave side where traction is apt to produce a transverse rupture. The forceps is gripped in the manner indicated so that the hand does not obscure the view. The hand of course is dropped below the level of the tibial head.

A certain amount of traction is necessary to keep the peripheral synovial attachment under tension as the blade of the curved knife is applied. This traction should be applied in the direction towards the midline of the joint rather than directly towards the operator. This ensures that the concave margin is not under tension with danger of rupture.

24

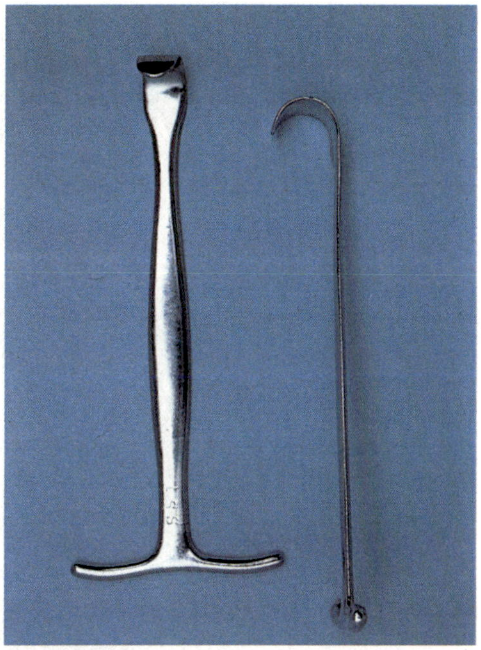

Use of retractors

24 **Retractors.** There is no exact point at which a description of the retractors should be interposed: they are used as soon as the skin incision is completed. On the other hand they only become essential when the joint cavity is entered. They are of sufficient importance to be illustrated and described individually rather than en masse. Although few in number they cover most circumstances likely to be encountered in the surgery of the menisci. First are simple conventional models of which two are required. The hand-hold is transverse in all of them thus eliminating the necessity to grip.

25

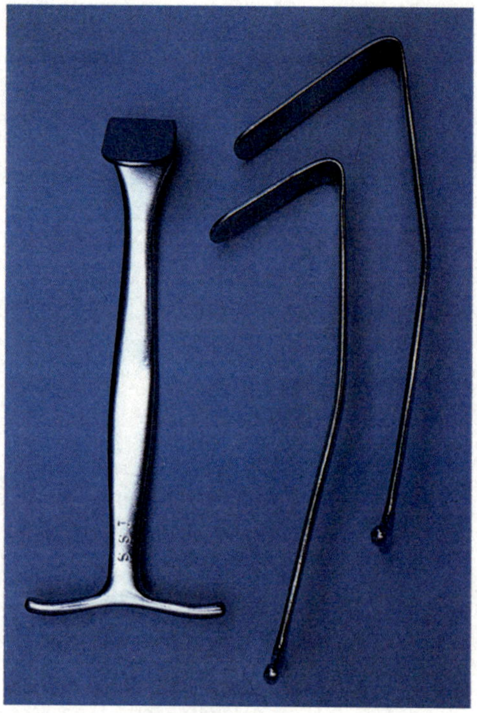

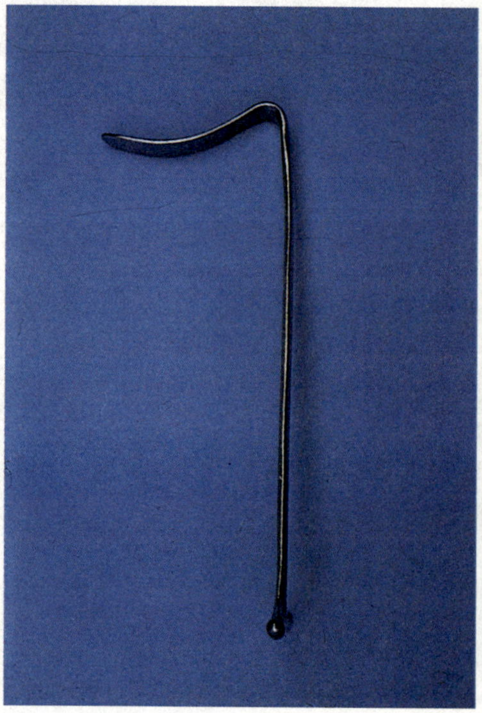

25 Retractors. The next three are wide-bladed (19mm) used in three lengths (32, 41 and 57mm) and used to retract the fat pad centrally in the variety of circumstances encountered. The angle in the shaft is 160 degrees and between shaft and blade 60 degrees.

26 Retractor. This instrument with a curved blade 10mm wide, is inserted between femoral condyle and collateral ligament when it is desirable to gain access to the periphery of the joint.

Dealing with effusion

27 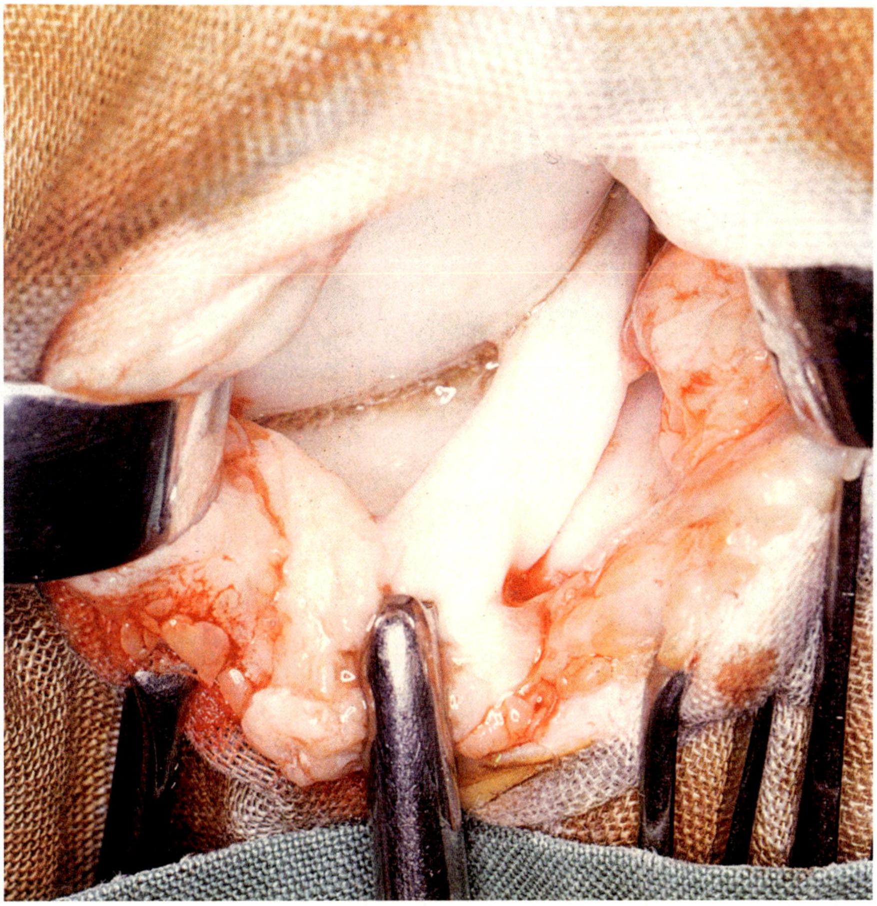

27 Dealing with effusion. When an effusion is present it is helpful if it is eliminated in its entirety at the commencement of the operation. This avoids passing dry swabs in and out of the joint throughout the procedure with consequent irritation of the synovial membrane and risk of postoperative effusion. With the joint in right-angled flexion the fluid will be lodged in the posterior compartment. With a small towel covering the gloved hand the fist is placed in the popliteal space, the fluid is pushed forward where it is removed by saline-moistened swabs or sucker.

28

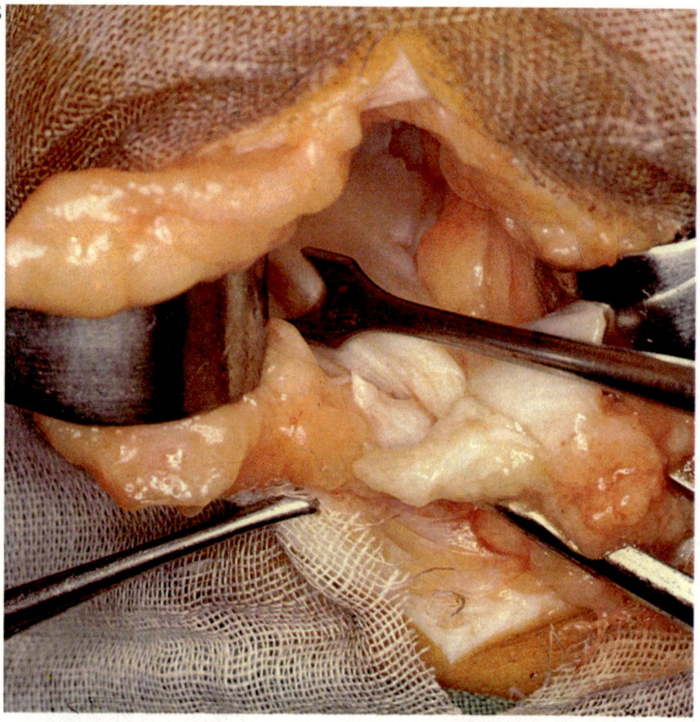

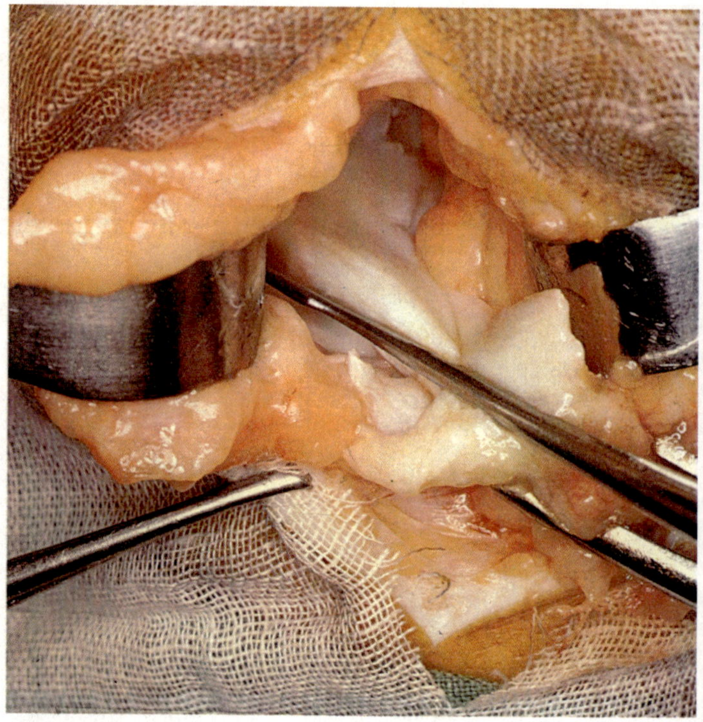

28 Use of curved knives in mobilising posterior half. Mode of use of curved knife in dividing the peripheral synovial attachments kept under tension by traction on the clamp. Note knife rotated 45 degrees towards centre of joint. (See **2**.)

29 Use of curved knives in mobilising posterior half. Alternatively the knife may be rotated 45 degrees towards the periphery. They are not held vertically and driven directly backwards into the joint.

30 Loss of orientation. If at any time, but particularly after the anterior half has been mobilised, there is a loss of orientation look under rather than on top of the meniscus to find your way.

30

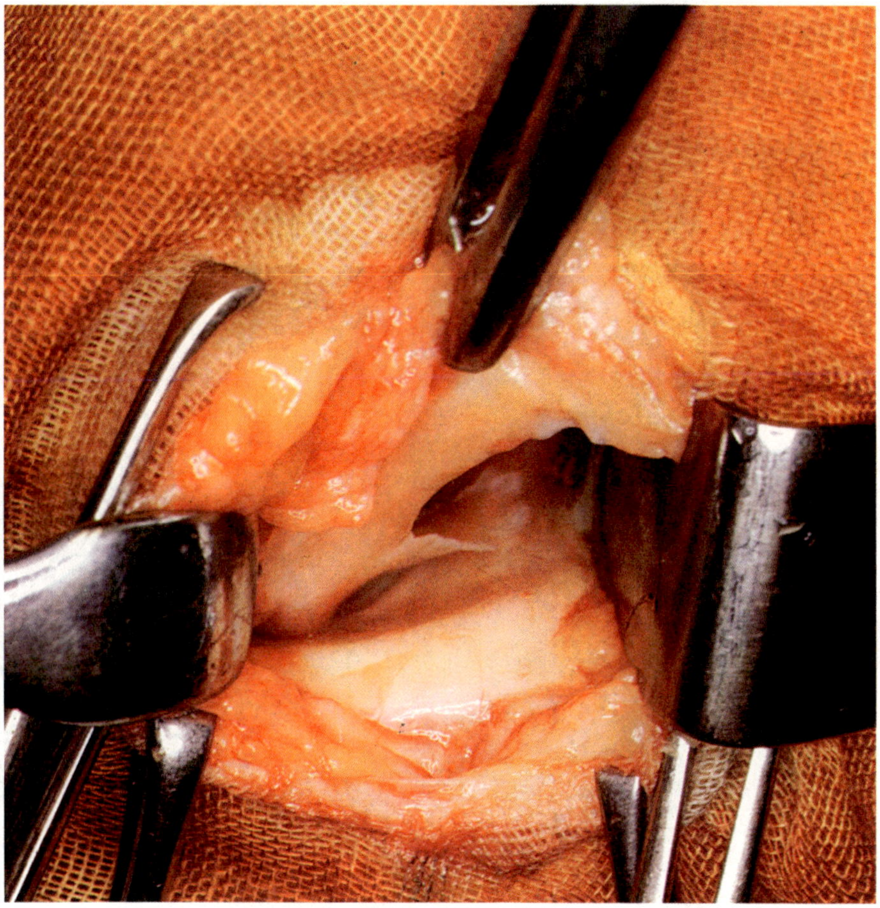

Effect of tibial rotation

31

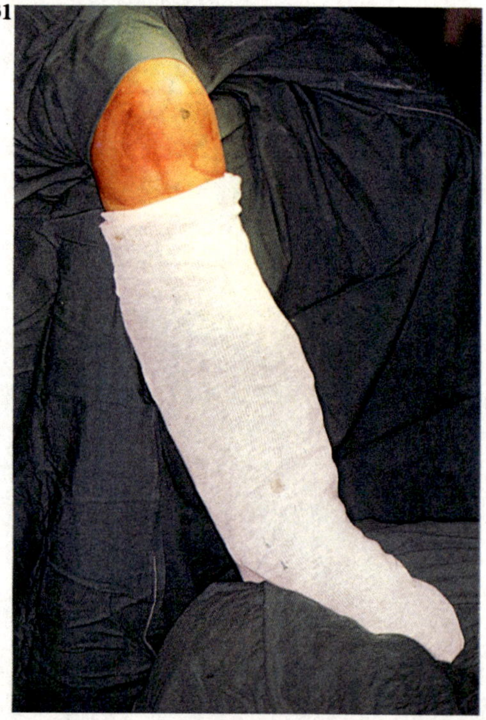

31 Effect of ability to rotate tibia. It is at this point of difficulty that the surgeon's knees, gripping the patient's foot, rotate the tibia laterally. This action, plus increasing the flexion of the knee, is quite remarkable in bringing the posterior synovial attachment within the compass of the curved knife.

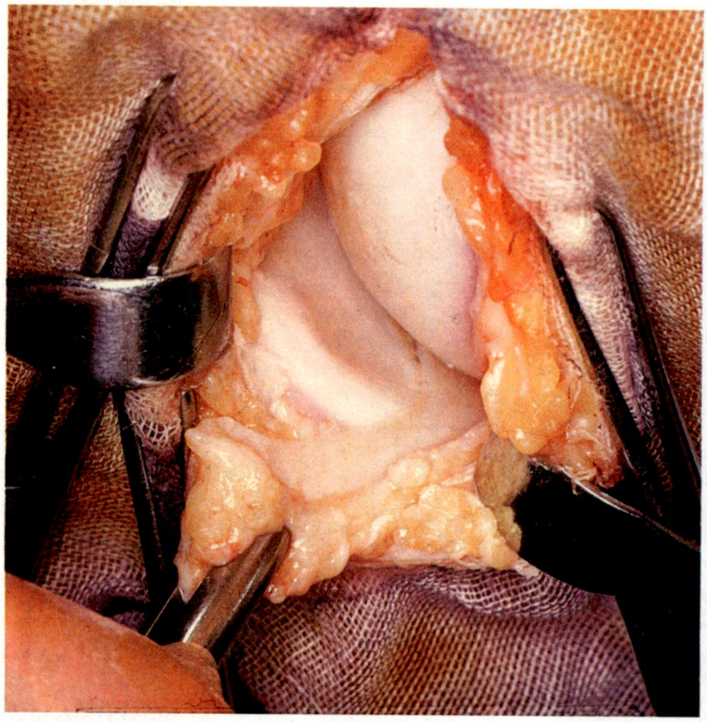

32 Effect of ability to rotate tibia. Note area of medial tibial head brought into view by lateral rotation of tibia.

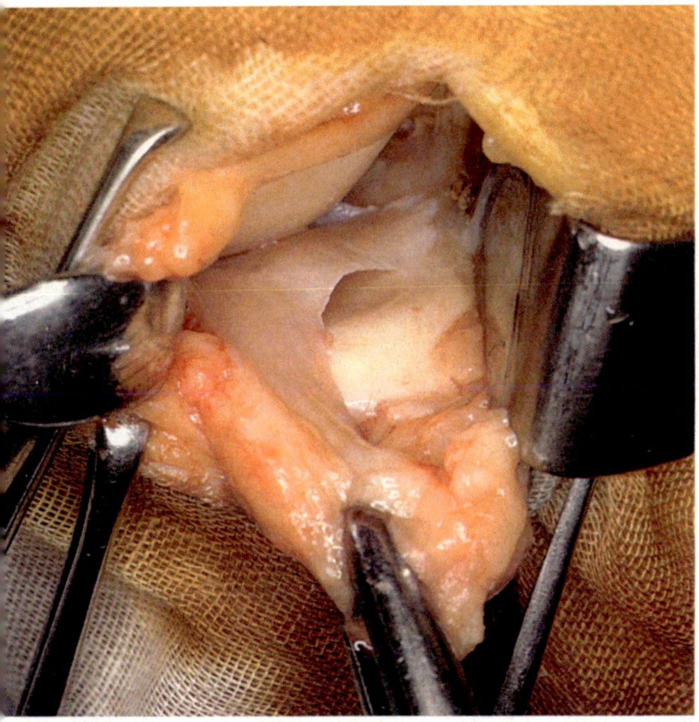

34

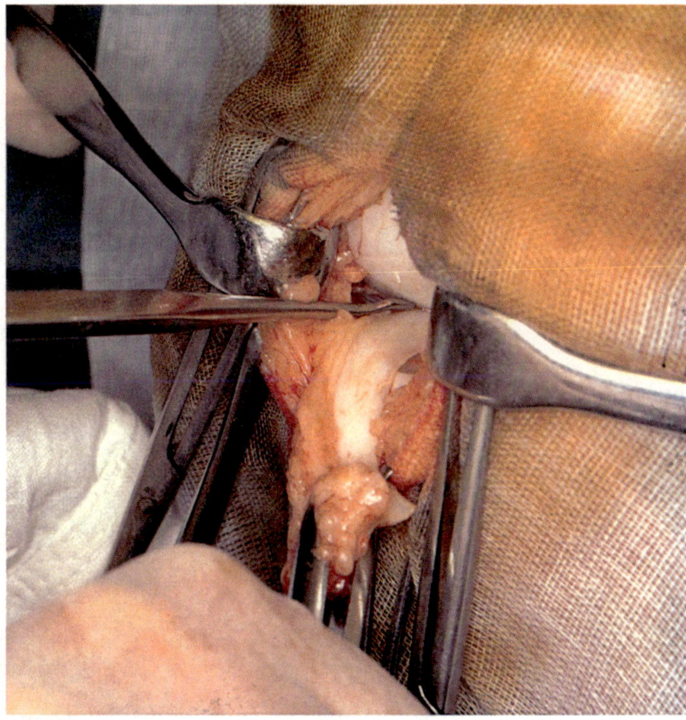

33 Effect of ability to rotate tibia. The posterior peripheral attachment is brought within the compass of the curved knife.

34 Effect of ability to rotate tibia. The curved knife, rotated 45 degrees towards the centre of the joint, follows the periphery of the meniscus towards the postero-central attachment.

35 The final move. The meniscus is displaced into the centre of the joint ready for division of the postero-central attachment in the manner indicated in (**4**). Note retractor (**24**) at periphery. Retractor (**25**) at fat pad and giving wide view of interior of joint. Note meniscus clamp (**22**) attached to periphery of anterior extremity and dropped below level of tibial table where it does not obstruct vision.

35

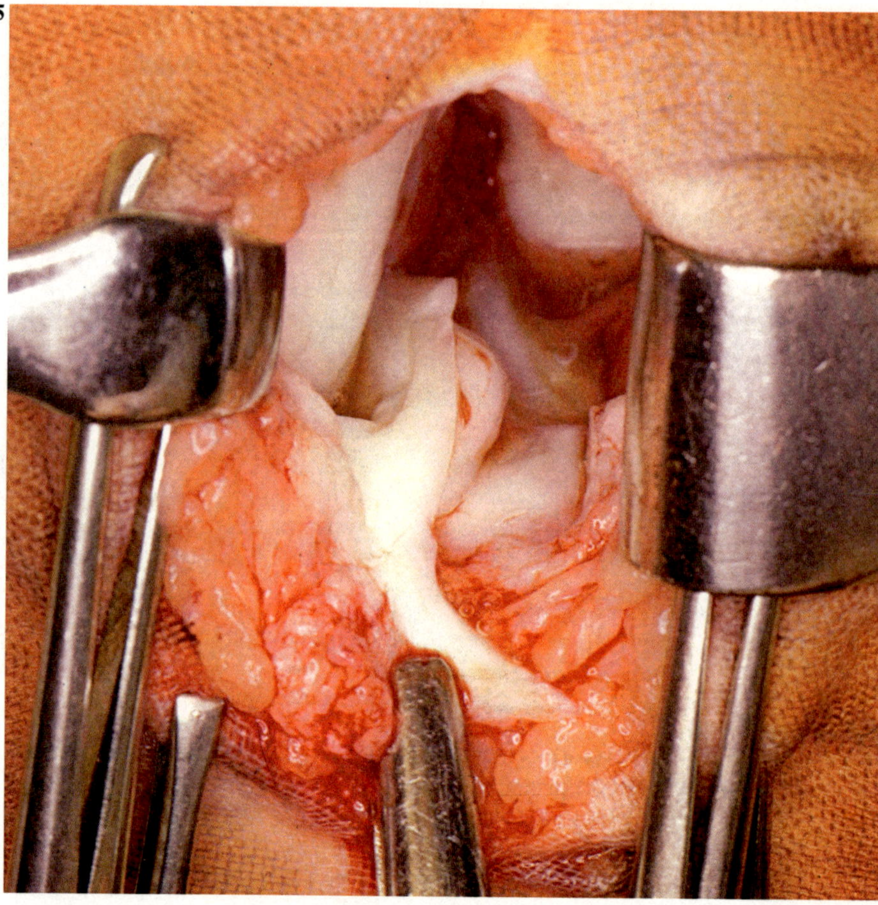

Excising torn meniscus

36

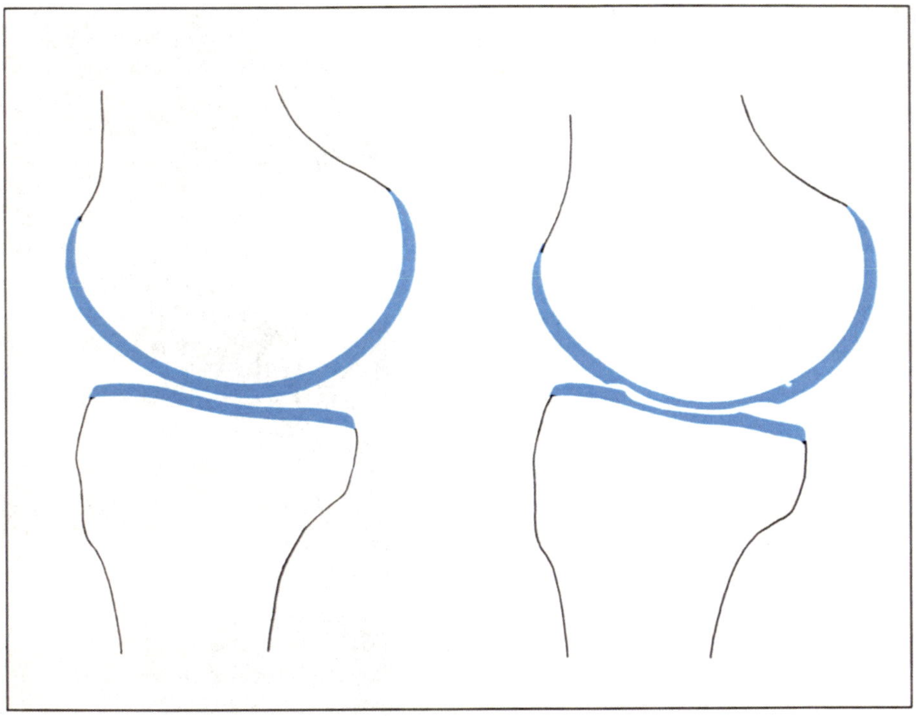

36 Excising torn meniscus from worn joint. It will be recognised that the knee does not wear evenly throughout the entire range of flexion but in the weight-bearing arc.

37 Excising torn meniscus from worn joint. In a joint as worn as this little space exists in the weight-bearing arc.

37

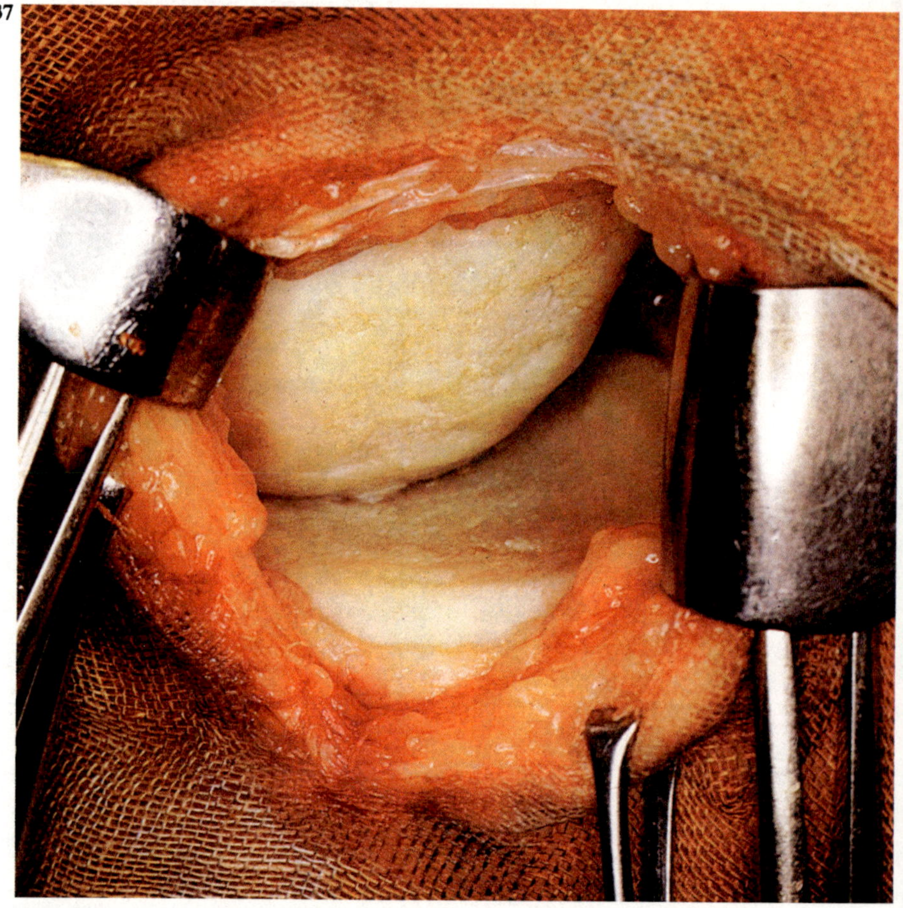

38

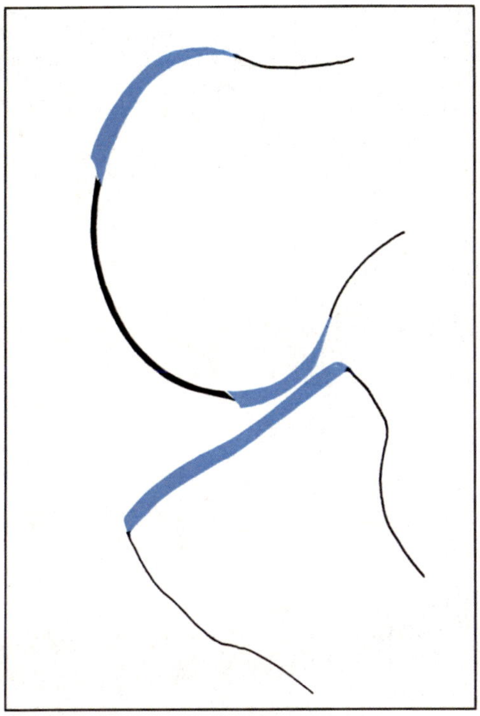

39

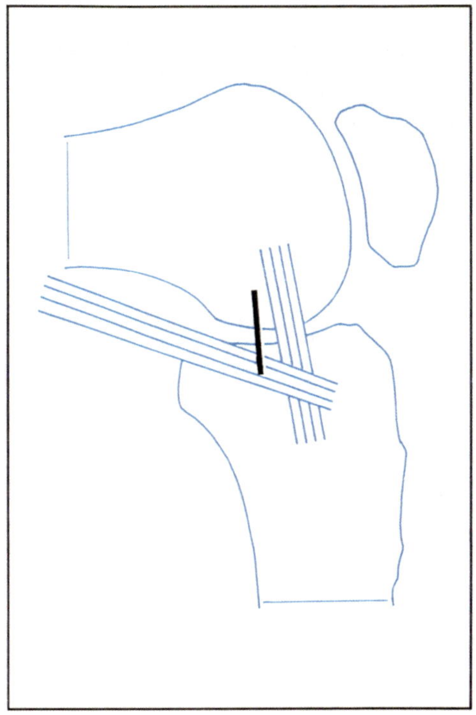

38 Excising torn meniscus from worn joint. In the difficult circumstances of removing a meniscus with a horizontal cleavage lesion from a worn joint, the posterior unworn part of the femoral condyle can be used in increasing the space available by hyperflexion of the knees. This is the reason for the necessity to have an operating table which will permit hyperflexion.

39 Situations demanding additional posterior incision. A second incision, of the size and site indicated, is required if accidental rupture of the meniscus takes place during the operation leaving a mobile posterior segment within the weight-bearing arc, and in failure to mobilise the posterior half through the anterior incision.

Posterior incision site

40 Site of posterior incision. To locate the site of the posterior incision curved mosquito forceps is entered along the joint line, whereby the point indicates the centre of the incision.

40

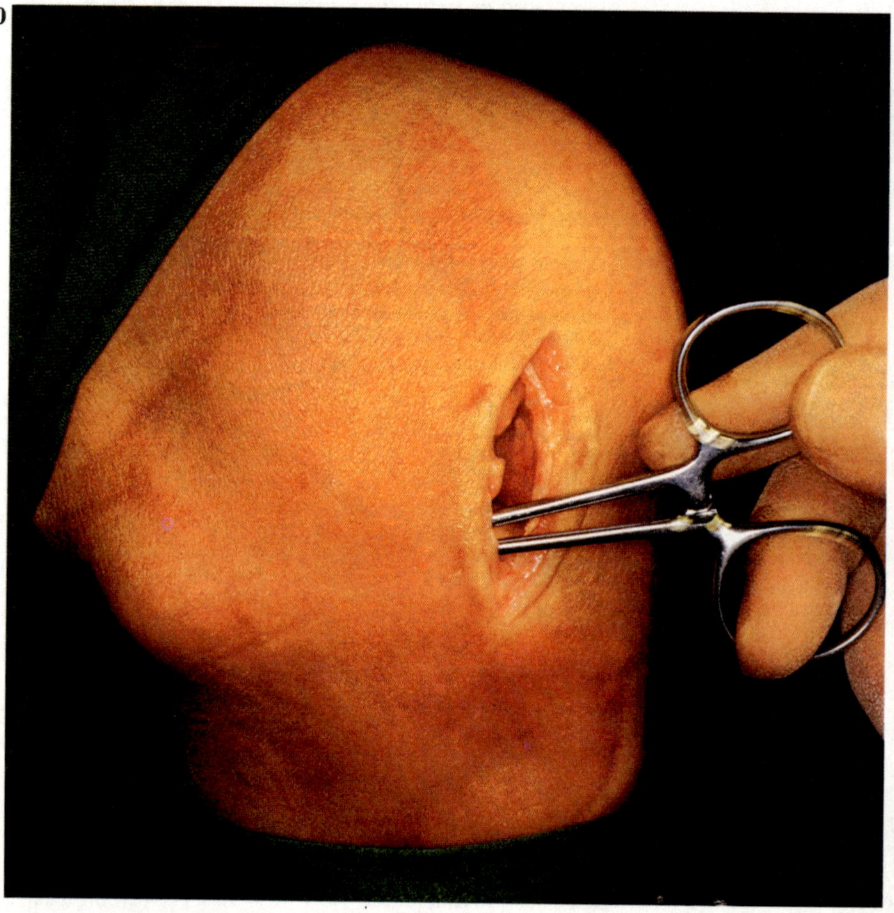

41 Site of posterior incision. The saphenous vein should be avoided. It will, of course, be empty under the control of the tourniquet. The capsule is divided in the line of the skin incision, the periphery of the meniscus located and separated from the capsule with one of the curved knives. The postero-central attachment is divided through the anterior incision again using one of the curved knives.

41

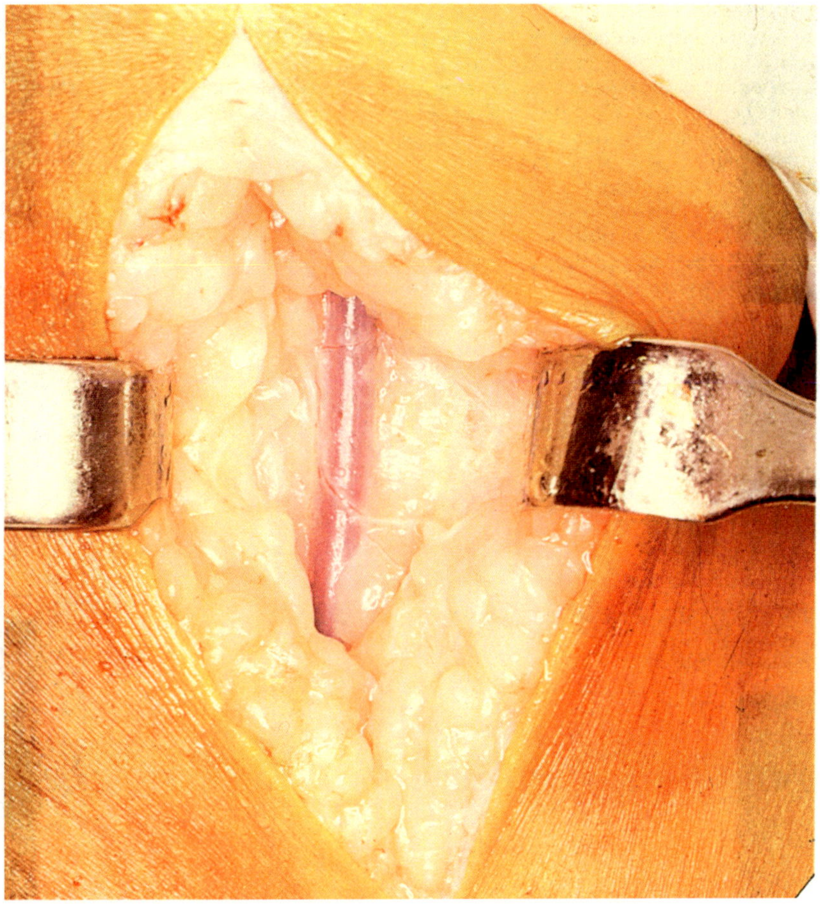

Second incision site

42 Situations demanding second incision: retained posterior segment. If, in circumstances of inadequate surgery, open or arthroscopic, the posterior half of the meniscus has been retained and is causing symptoms it must be removed. Operation cannot be performed through a single anterior incision: the junction between the regenerated anterior segment and the retained posterior segment is weak and will not permit traction to be exerted. In such circumstances the regenerated portion is mobilised through the anterior incision and the retained posterior segment mobilised through the posterior incision as described. The operator then returns to the anterior incision for division of the postero-central attachment.

42

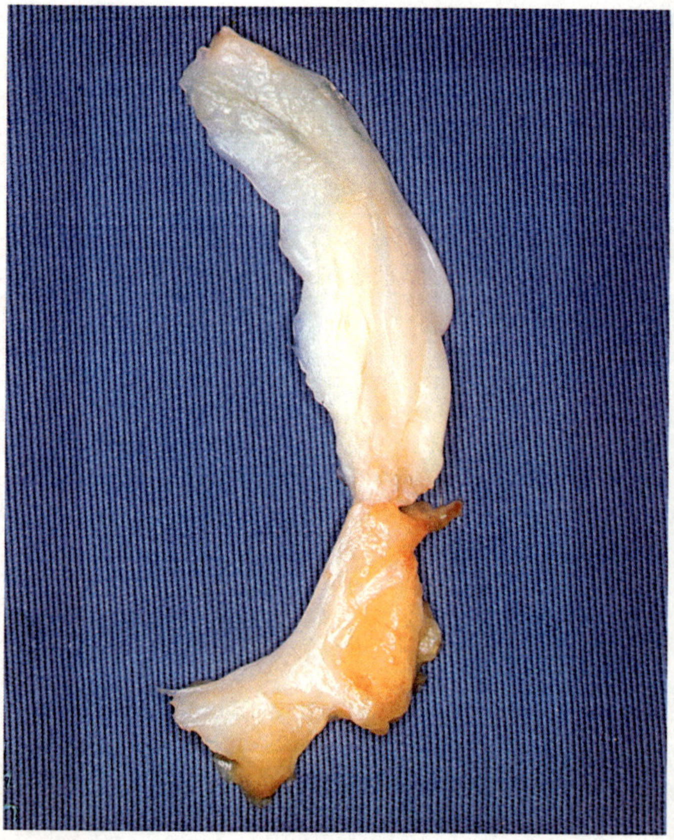

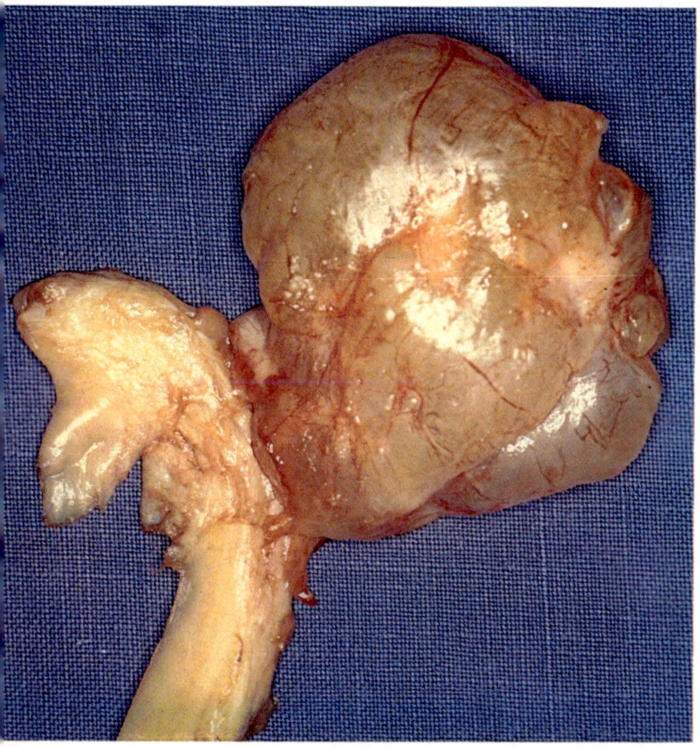

43 Other situations demanding second incision. The circumstances of cystic degeneration of the posterior segment of the medial meniscus with symptoms suggesting that the meniscus is torn demand that the posterior incision, to mobilise and identify the cyst, is made initially. The anterior incision is added to mobilise the anterior two-thirds of the meniscus.

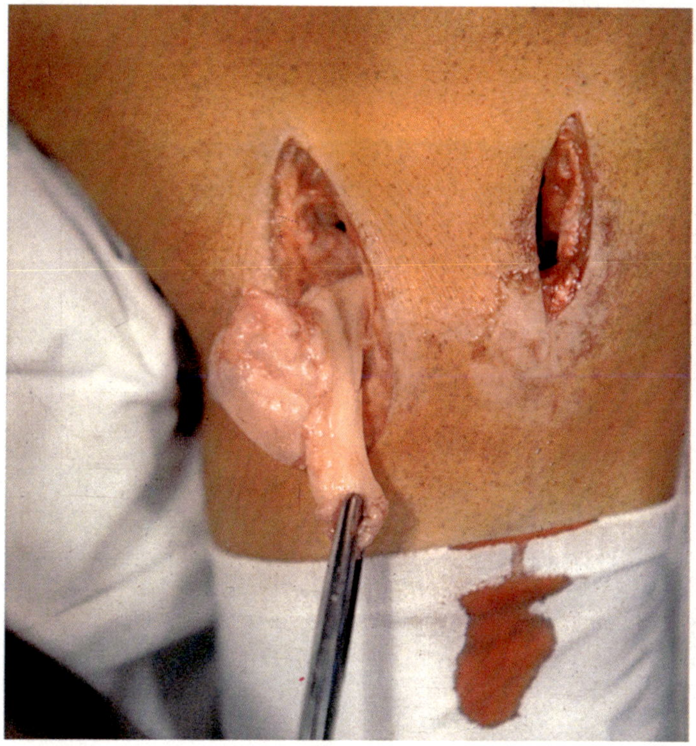

44 Other situations demanding second incision. In cystic degeneration of the posterior segment of the medial meniscus the cyst together with attached meniscus is eventually presented through the posterior incision before the central fixation is divided.

Cystic degeneration

45
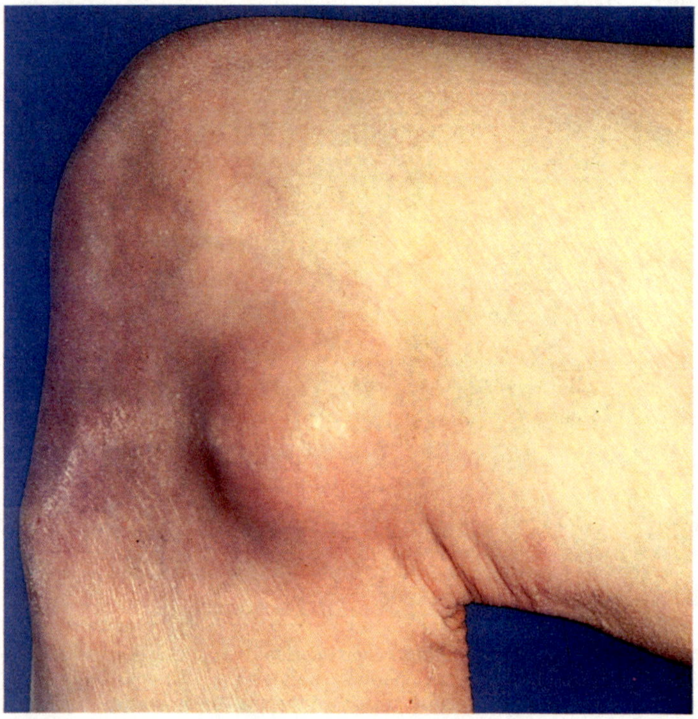

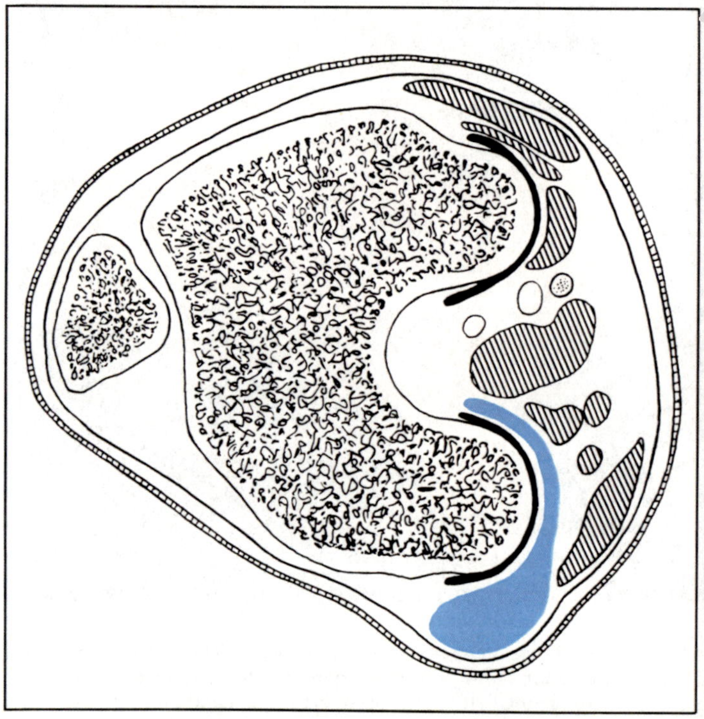

45 Cystic degeneration posterior segment medial meniscus. But the cyst must be positively identified as arising in the meniscus lest a normal meniscus be excised in error.

46 Cystic degeneration posterior segment medial meniscus: differential diagnosis. A popliteal cyst (gastrocnemio-semimembranosus bursa) sometimes presents on the medial joint line posteriorly producing a swelling similar to cystic degeneration.

Rupture of lateral meniscus

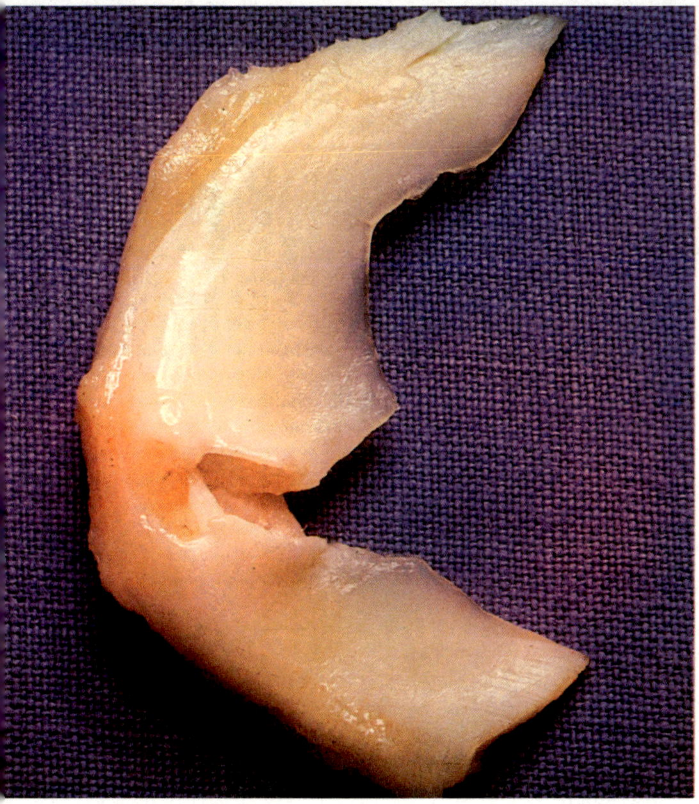

47 **No additional incision is necessary on lateral side.** On the lateral side rupture of a meniscus, the site of a parrot-beak tear, is common leaving the posterior two-thirds of the meniscus requiring to be removed. In contrast to the medial side a second incision is never necessary.

48

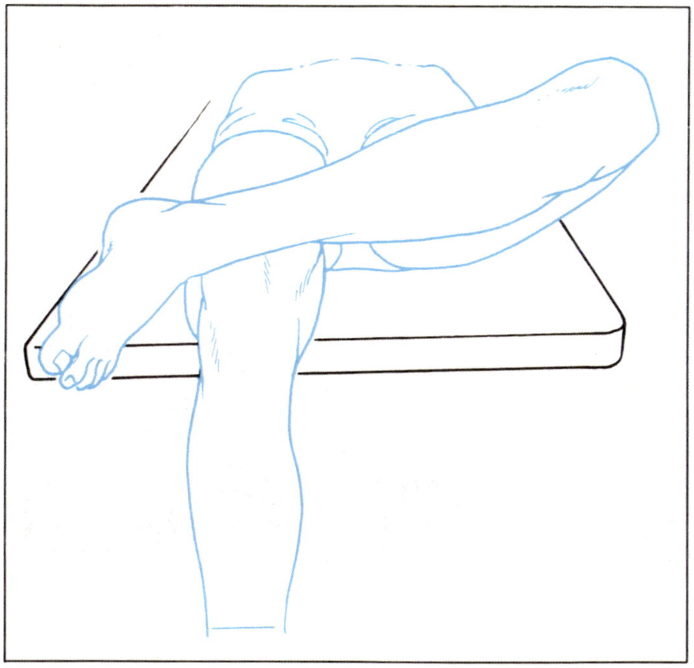

48 Access to lateral compartment. If the hip is flexed and rotated laterally so that the lateral aspect of the ankle rests on the suprapatellar region of the other knee the joint is in maximum varus angulation in maximum lateral rotation. In this position a wide gap exists between femur and tibia.

49

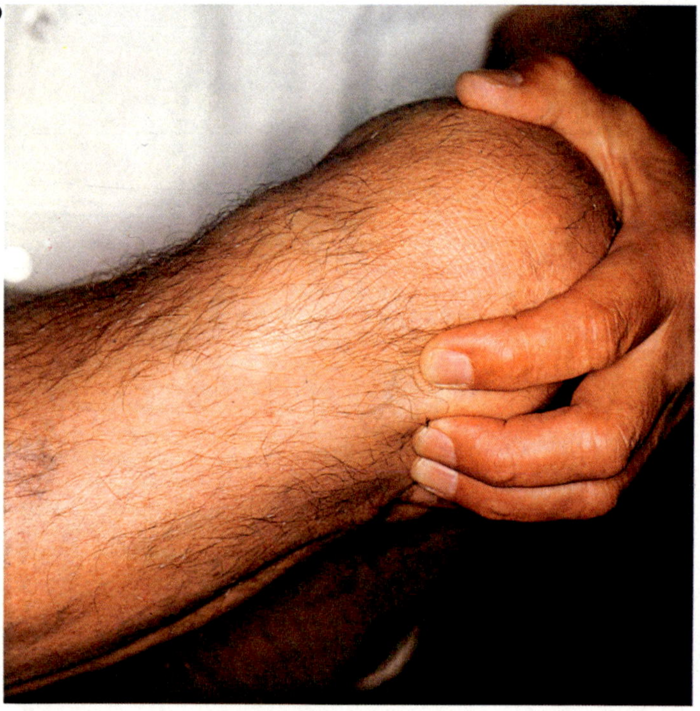

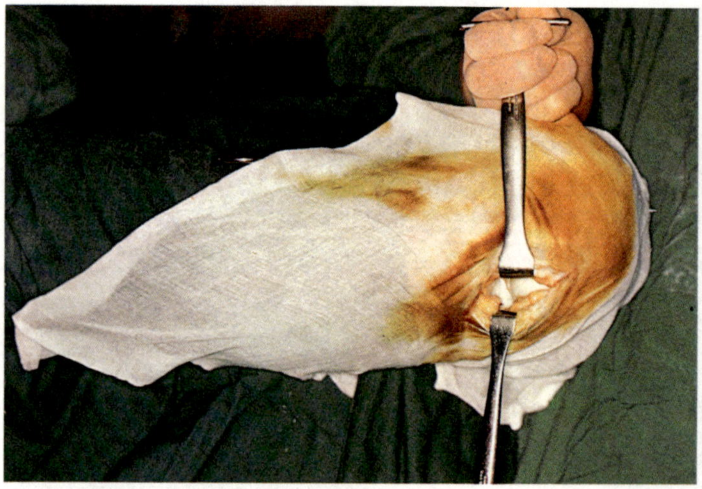

50 Access to lateral compartment. To reach the postero-lateral aspect of the joint the retractors in the limited vertical incision remain in position held by an assistant. The knee is flexed to a right angle and rotated into the position shown in (**48**) and (**49**). The incision is now horizontal in the eyes of the surgeon.

49 Access to lateral compartment: the position demonstrated. The tips of the forefinger and long finger have been entered in the gap. Between the two is the ilio-tibial band.

51 Access to lateral compartment. Note the remarkable exposure provided by this manoeuvre. In this example the posterior half of the meniscus has been removed. The structure seen is the posterior capsule.

51

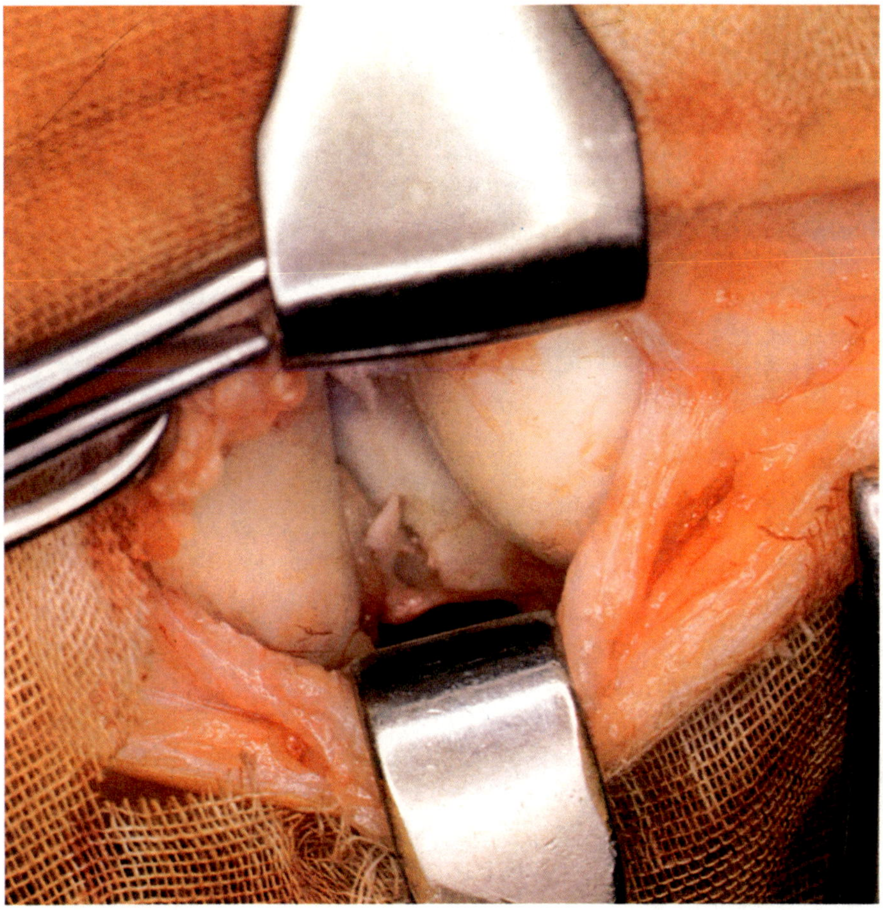

Termination of operation

52A Closing the incision. Interrupted sutures are used. They are inserted in a special way to avoid showing catgut within the joint, thought to be a cause of postoperative effusion: the needle picks up the capsule, then picks up the synovial membrane in such a manner so that the suture does not appear within the joint.

52a

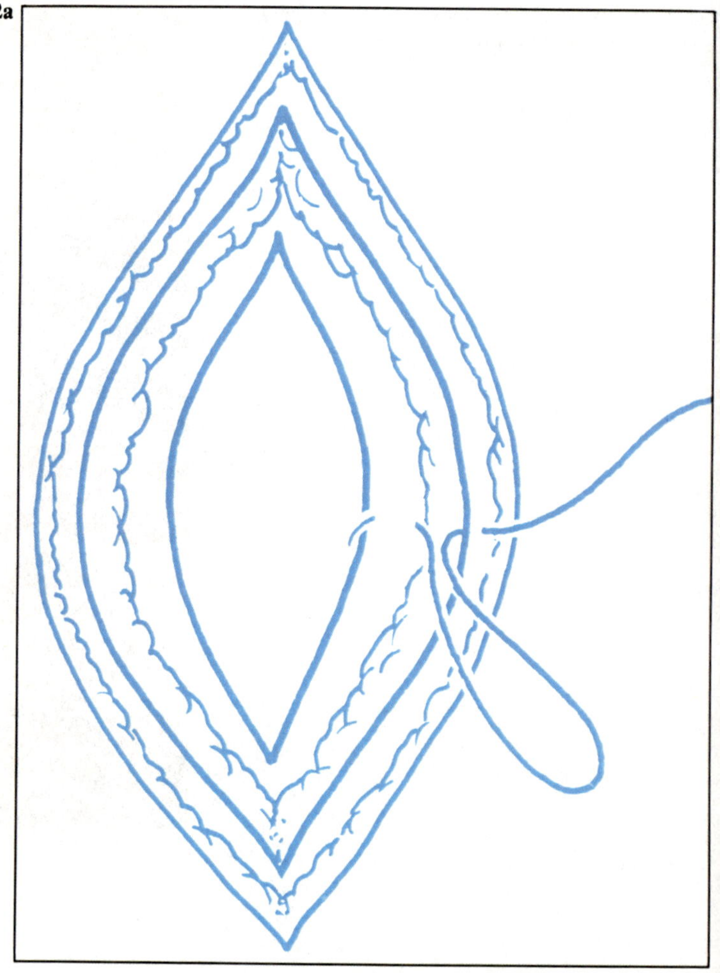

52 Termination of operation. In closing the skin the knee should be in the same degree of flexion as when the incision was made.

52

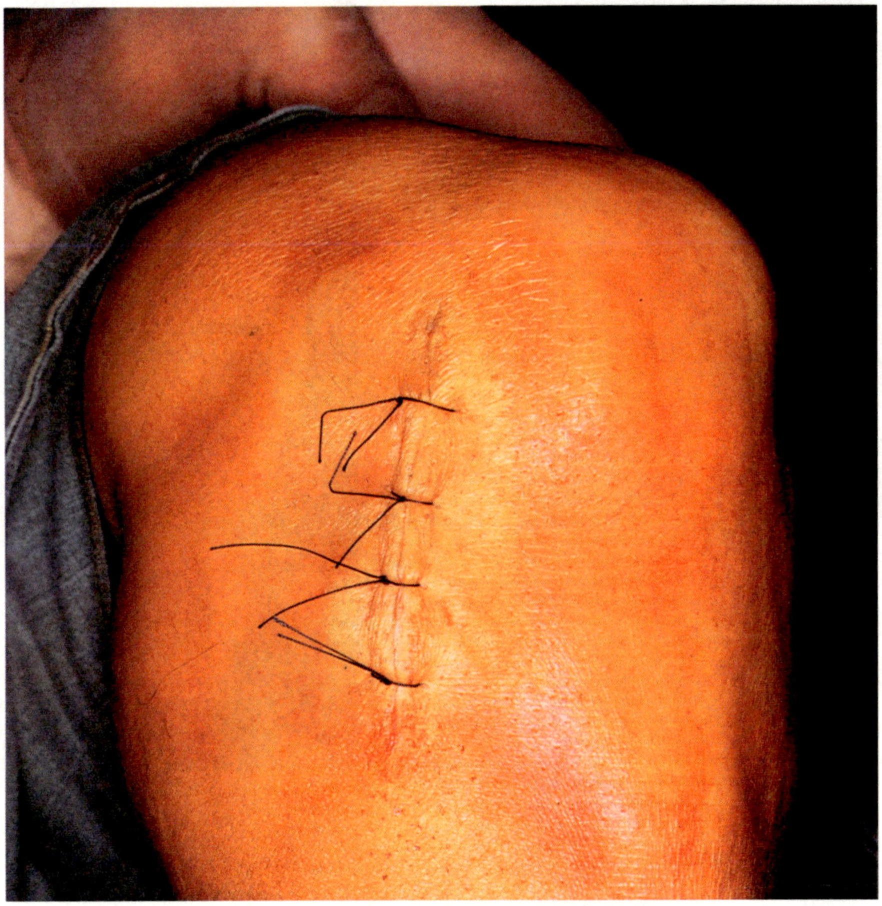

53 Termination of operation. At the end of the operation, and before the tourniquet is released, a compression, or Jones, bandage is applied to control capillary ooze from the divided synovial membrane at the periphery of the joint. It consists of three thick layers of sheet cottonwool of high quality in terms of elasticity and compressibility. Interposed between each layer are two layers of 15cm (6 inch) bandage of non-stretch material. A total of some 12 metres is required. The bandage should be applied by the surgeon who performs the operation; not by an inexperienced assistant. The completed bandage should have the consistency of a 'ripe melon'.

53

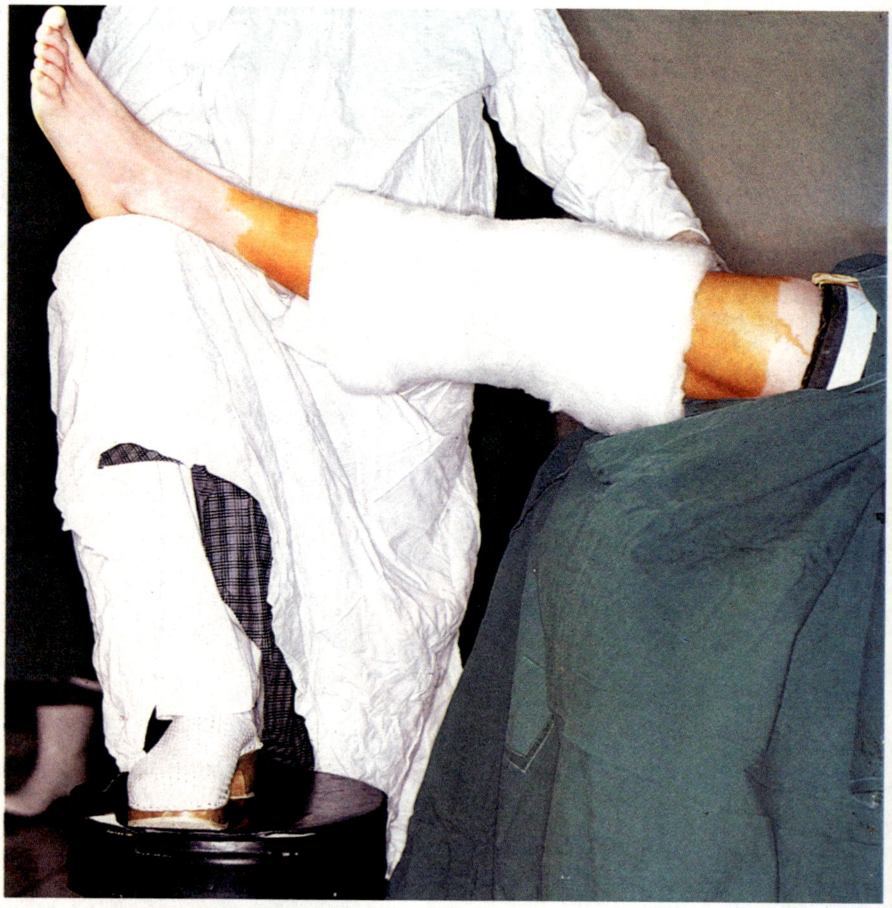

Exercise therapy

54

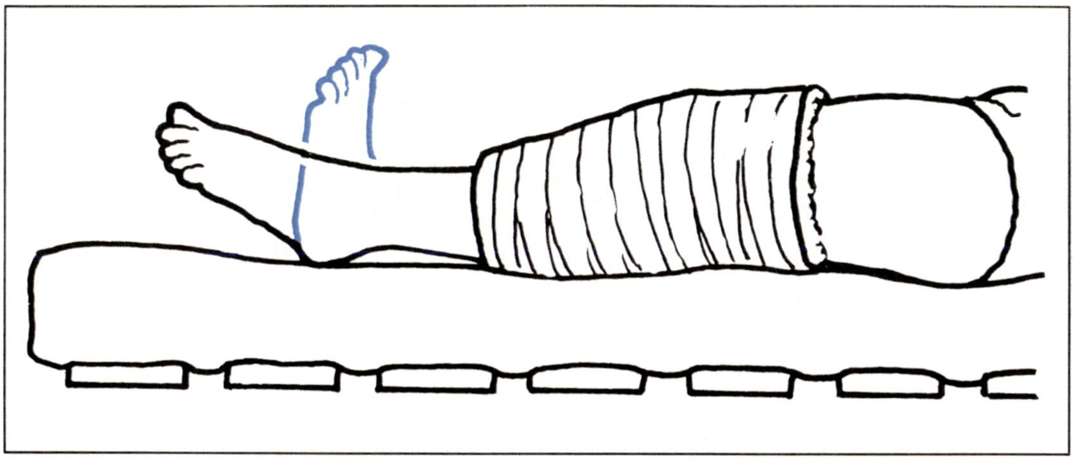

54 After treatment: exercise therapy. It will be indicated later that haemarthrosis is the most important common complication of the operation. It is for this reason that immediate quadriceps exercises are not advised. On the first three to four days patients practise hourly, or preferably more often, calf and anterior compartment exercises in the form of plantar and dorsiflexion of the foot. This is much in the interests of avoiding deep vein thrombosis but to some extent it slackens the compression bandage which the patient may feel tight. It has the advantage that it involves the patient in his own recovery at the earliest stage.

Note fracture-board bed. It is essential that the mattress is firm so that the patient can turn over without flexing the knee. A soft mattress is a source of pain in turning with the possible increased danger of haemarthrosis.

55

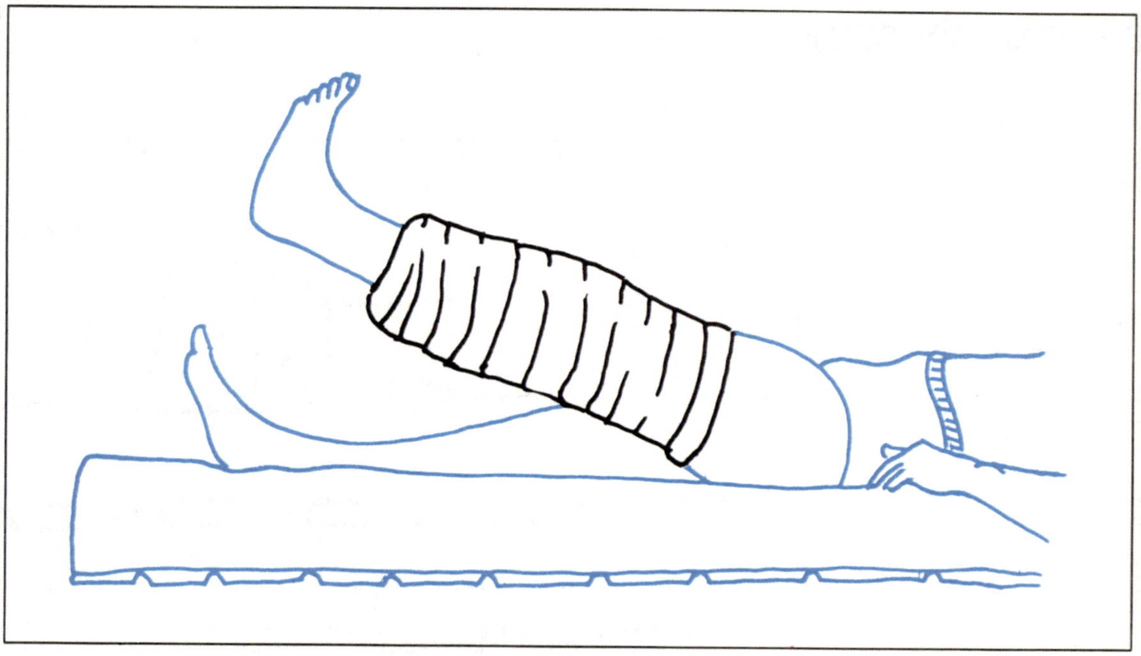

55 After treatment: exercise therapy. On the third or fourth day quadriceps exercises begin in the form of straight-leg raising. This is essential exercising in the simplest form not requiring the patient to learn anything new. It can with advantage be taught on the sound limb as soon as the patient has overcome the immediate effects of operation.

56

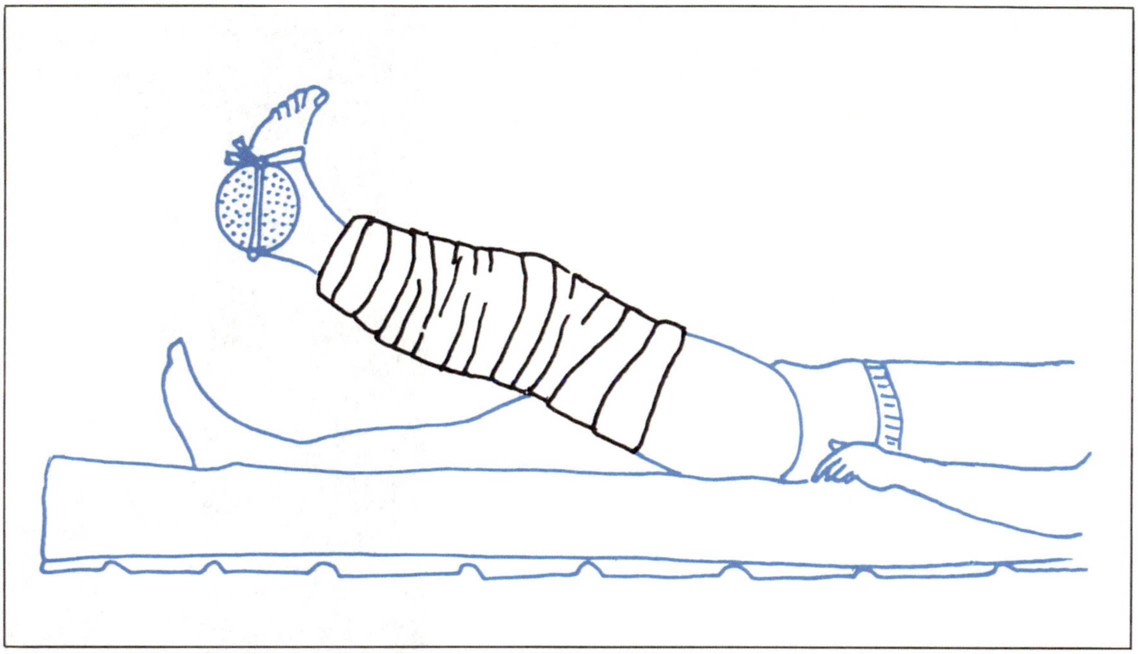

56 After treatment: exercise therapy. The next stage is to load the straight-leg raising, increasing the resistance to be overcome, by attaching a weight to the foot starting with a half to one kilogram and increasing, depending on progress, to two to four kilograms.

57 Resumption of weightbearing. When weightbearing is resumed on, say, the tenth day when the skin stitches are removed, a normal heel-and-toe gait is taught. A single stick (cane) is not permitted. The compression bandage is retained. It possibly prevents effusion but in any event gives a sense of security. The patient is permitted to walk short distances and then to sit. To stand about is to induce effusion.

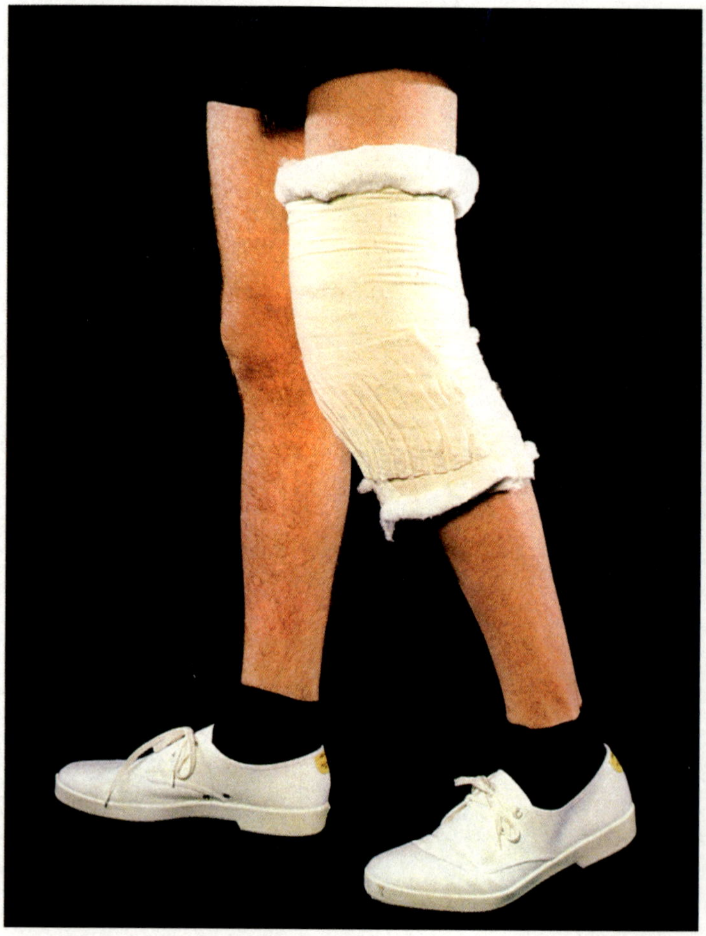

Haemarthrosis

58 Complications: haemarthrosis. Transient pain localised to the site of operation is to be expected on commencing exercise therapy in the form of straight-leg raising and quadriceps drill. Persistent severe pain results from some local cause and warrants investigation. It is usually caused by haematoma between: 1 Skin and capsule; 2 Capsule and synovial membrane; or 3, most important of all, within the joint in the form of a haemarthrosis. 1 And 2 are usually caused by failure to ligate or coagulate sizeable vessels. The treatment is evacuation of the clot under strict aseptic precautions. 3 Is caused by either capillary ooze and necessitates no more than aspiration and the re-application of the compression bandage, or, more uncommon, but much more important, haemorrhage from a sizeable artery.

58

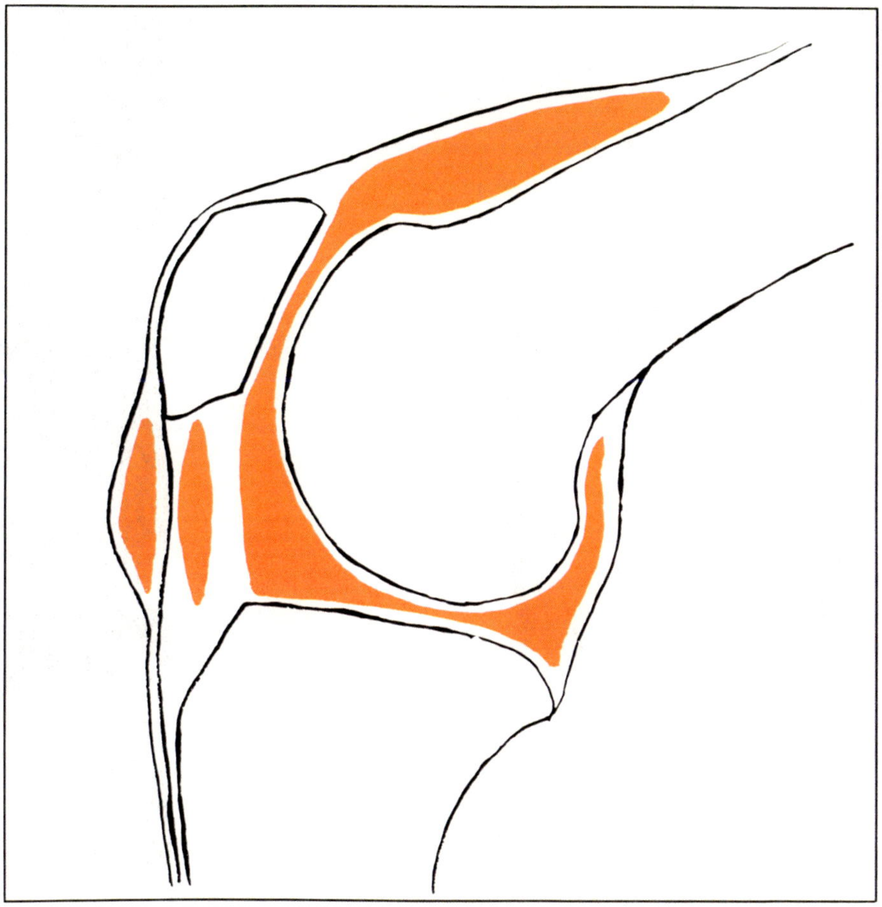

59

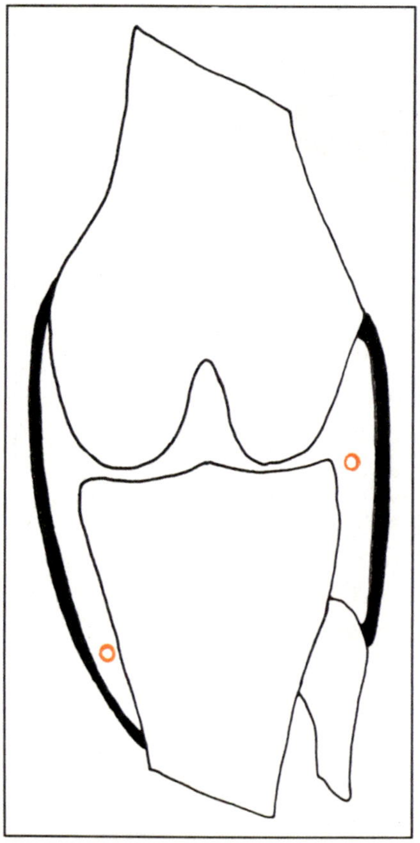

59 Haemarthrosis of arterial origin. The inferior medial geniculate artery lies well below the joint line and should not be divided at operation. The inferior lateral geniculate artery is located at the periphery of the meniscus and is almost invariably divided at operation.

60

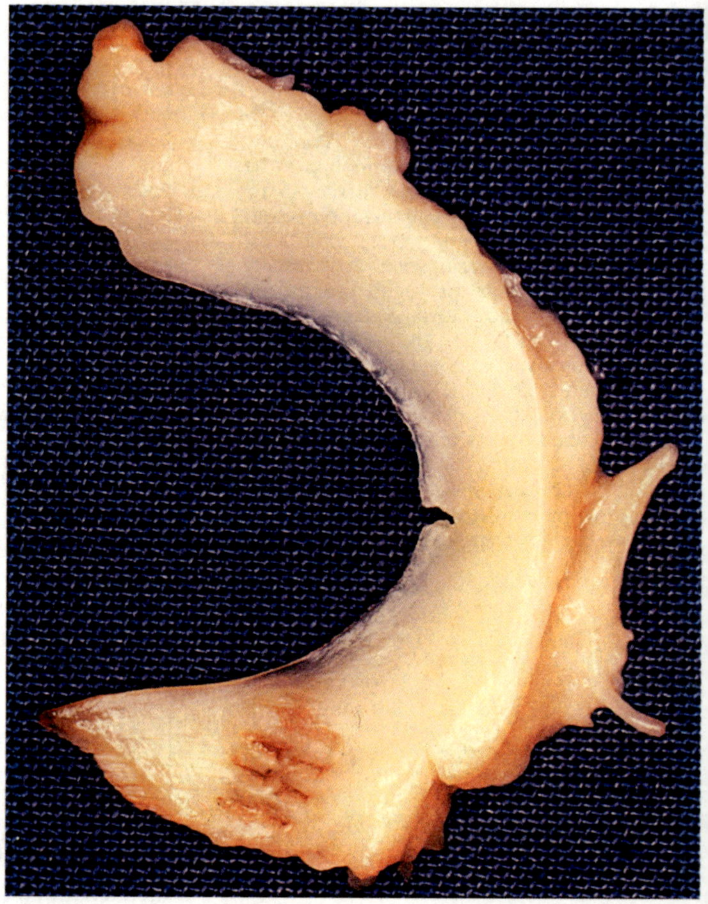

60 Haemarthrosis of arterial origin. Lateral meniscus of normal conformation to show section of inferior lateral geniculate artery. No haemarthrosis resulted from division of the artery.

61 Haemarthrosis of arterial origin. In a large congenital discoid lateral meniscus the geniculate artery may be of even greater dimensions. No haemarthrosis resulted from division of the artery.

61

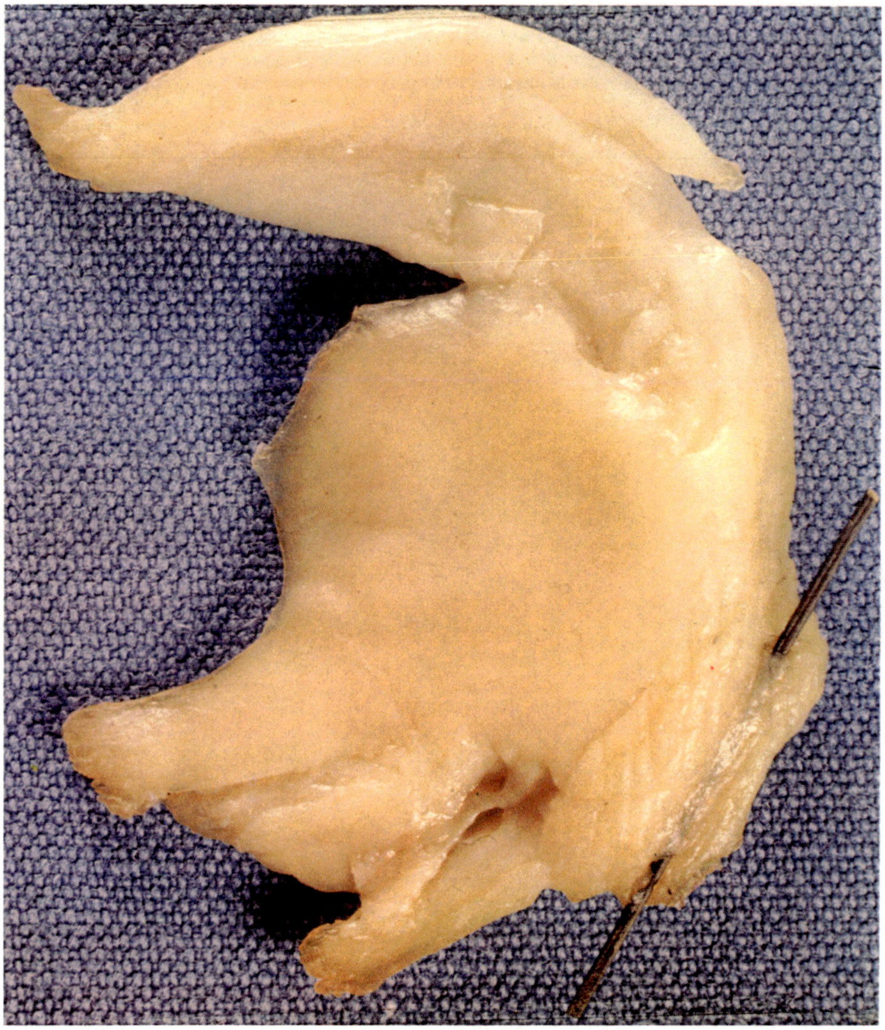

62 Haemarthrosis of arterial origin. If the inferior lateral geniculate artery is divided as in **60** and **61**, the ends retract and no harm results. It is when incomplete division occurs, such as a slice out of the wall, that the danger of a pulsating haemarthrosis occurs.

62

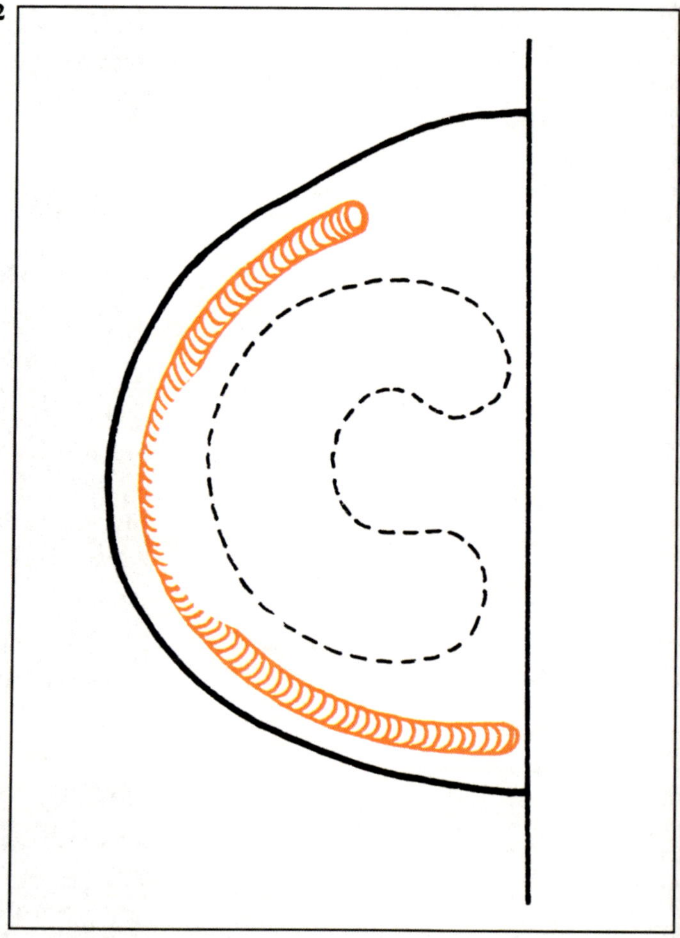

63 Haemarthrosis of arterial origin: securing haemostasis. If this complication is uncommon when it does occur it poses the impossible problem of finding the bleeding point. A suture on a round-bodied needle, entered blindly at the joint line, readily stops the bleeding.

63

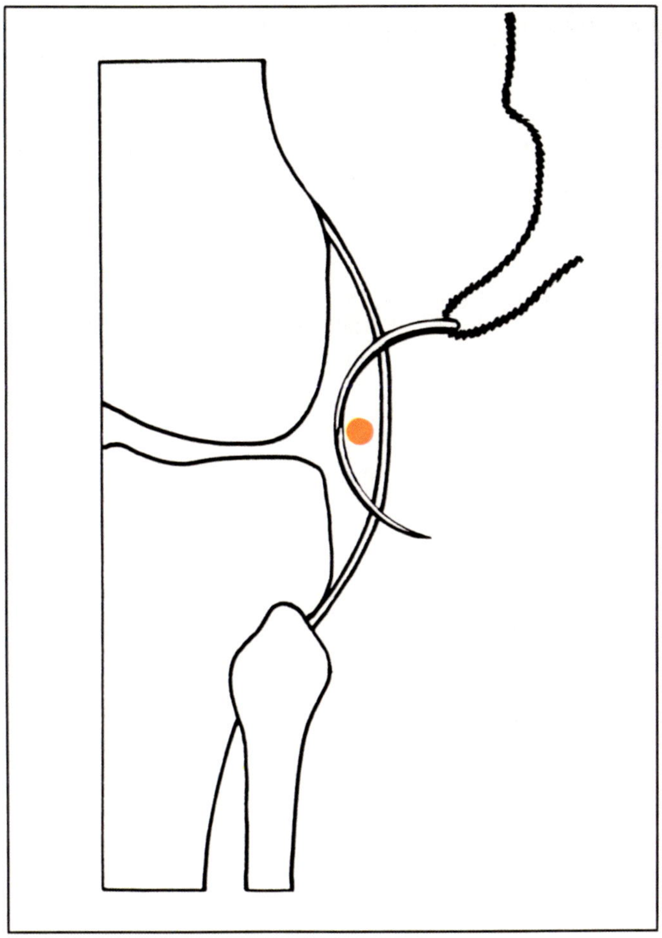

Patellar plexus injury

64 Complications: injury to patellar plexus. The superficial sensory nerves which make up the patellar plexus seem particularly sensitive to injury. The saphenous nerve pierces the deep fascia on the medial side between the tendons of sartorius and gracilis. Before doing so it gives off the infrapatellar branch which passes forward about a finger's breadth below the joint line to form the patellar plexus in association with branches of the medial, lateral and intermediate cutaneous nerves. Some of the branches are invariably cut in knee incisions leading to temporary areas of anaesthesia.

64

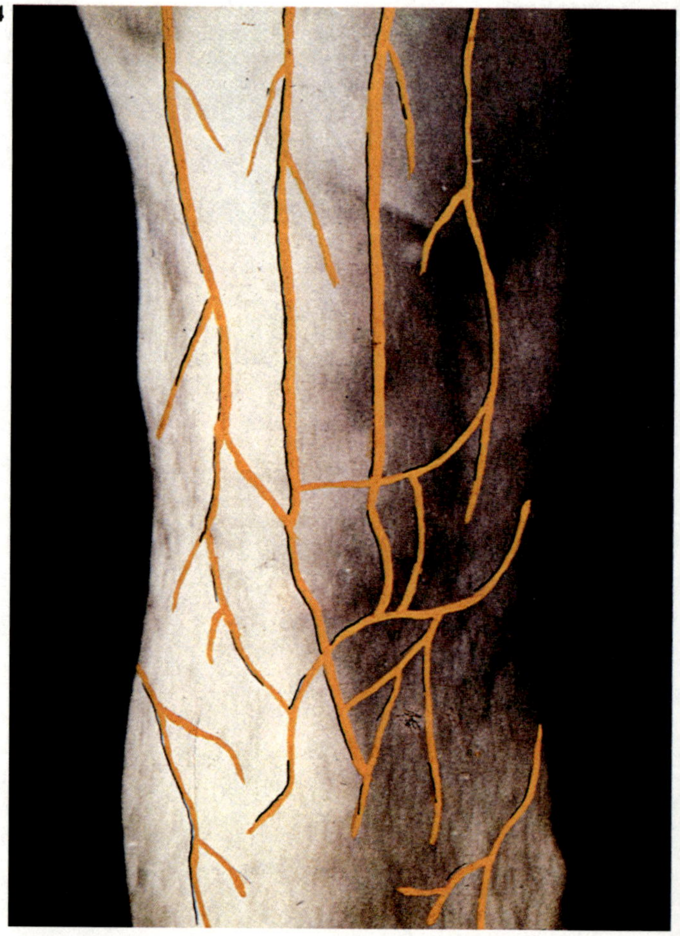

65 Complications: neuroma of infrapatellar branch of saphenous nerve. It has been indicated that an incision on the medial side of the joint should not extend more than a finger's breadth below the joint line. Anatomy is not an exact science: the nerve must frequently be cut without undue consequences. When a neuroma occurs following meniscectomy it is probably because the nerve has been wounded, rather than cut, and becomes adherent to the scar.

When this complication occurs the scar is excised, the neuroma isolated and the nerve traced in a proximal direction and divided with a sharp scalpel. This measure ensures that a further neuroma is not adherent to the cutaneous scar.

65

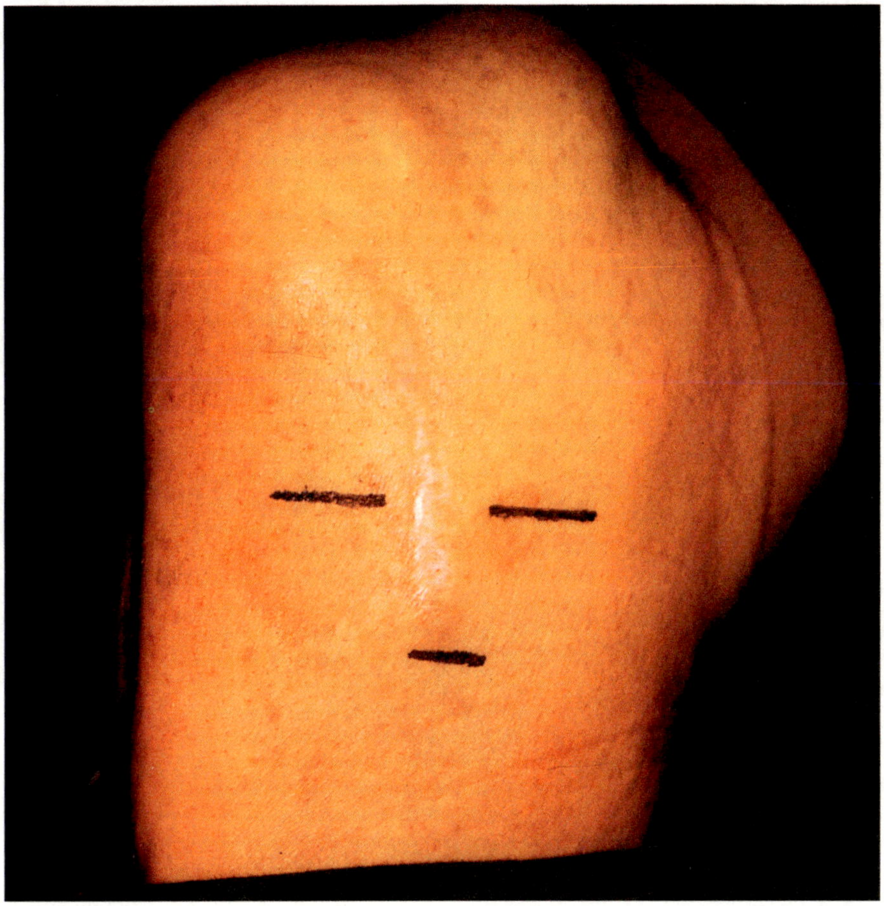

Reference and further reading

Smillie, I.S., *Injuries of the Knee Joint* (5th edition). Churchill Livingstone, Edinburgh, London & New York, 1978.

Index

Numbers in medium type refer to page numbers; those in **bold** refer to figure and caption numbers.